THE PATH TO SLEEP

Exercises for an Ancient Skill

Hypnotic Training in the Neurology
Psychology & Physiology of Sleep

•

Lincoln Stoller, PhD, CHt

MindStrengthBalance.com

Also by Lincoln Stoller:
The Learning Project, Rites of Passage, 2019
Becoming Lucid, Self-Awareness in Sleeping & Waking Life, 2019

First Edition.
Published 2019 by Mind Strength Balance
Victoria, British Columbia, Canada
https://www.mindstrengthbalance.com

Copyright © 2019 Lincoln Stoller, All rights reserved.

Except for brief excerpts in reviews, no part of this book may be reproduced in any form, or by any means, electronic or mechanical, including photocopying, recording, or by any information storage and retrieval system, without the written permission of the publisher.

Stoller, Lincoln, 1956- author.
the path to sleep : exercises for an ancient skill / Lincoln Stoller.
ISBN 978-1-9992538-1-3 (mobi) | ISBN 978-1-9992538-2-0 (epub)
ISBN 978-1-9992538-0-6 (paper) | ISBN 978-1-9992538-3-7 (hard cover)
ISBN 978-1-9992538-4-4 (audio)
Subjects: LCSH: Awareness. | Dreams. | Mental suggestion. | Sleep.

Cover Photo:
Lasse Holst Hansen

DISCLAIMER:

This book is designed to provide information on the subject matter provided. It is sold with the understanding that the author does not provide medical advice or treatment. If medical assistance is required, the services of a licensed professional should be sought. The purpose of this book is to educate and inform. The publisher, author or any other dealer or distributor shall not be held liable to the purchaser or any other person or entity with respect to any liability, loss, or damage caused or alleged to be caused directly or indirectly by this book.

Praise for *The Path to Sleep*

"This book is not just a book, it's a hands-on guide to the root cause of all those sleepless nights. It offers a complete paradigm shift to transform the very context of insomnia from something to survive to something to celebrate for its unique ability to act as a catalyst for growth."
— **Mollie McGlocklin**, author and host of www.sleepisaskill.com.

"The Path To Sleep is the first systematic application of hypnosis to sleep dysfunction despite ample evidence of hypnosis's remarkable positive effect. The book's hypnotic audio files address problems of rumination, emotional and physical stress, brain rhythms, sleep hygiene, and dreams. This is much needed non-pharmaceutical guidance for those with all forms of insomnia, and will be of special benefit to the elderly."
— **Dr. Robert S. Rosenberg**, author of *Sleep Soundly Every Night, Feel Fantastic Every Day*, and *The Doctor's Guide to Sleep Solutions for Stress & Anxiety*.

"If you're that person who just can't sleep, no matter what—even drugs aren't doing such a great job—READ THIS BOOK! From the opening pages of The Path to Sleep, *you will quickly get the personality, the passion, and the compassion of Lincoln Stoller. Yeah, sure, there are many sleep experts and science-based facts on the internet, and herbs and potions and chanting. How's all that working for you so far? Lincoln nails it by staying steadfast with the bottom line. Sleep is not the problem. You are."*
— **Sandy Ames, CHt**, author of *Sleep Now!: Self Hypnosis Meditation*.

"The Path to Sleep is a transformation into a new mind. It will require you to open yourself up to new ideas, to challenge long-held beliefs and to reach for your life. If you ever needed to believe in 'miracles' but needed some science to bring some clarity to your hopes, then this is a book for you."
— **Krystalle Lebray**, Fitness Coach and Kinesiologist.

"I just love the audio files. Haven't slept this great in a while, and the dreams have been really crazy. Wish I could understand what they are telling me."
— **Robert L.**, working with my book *Becoming Lucid*.

"I can say without doubt: my sleep has improved a lot. I can fall asleep faster with much fewer days lying in bed trying to fall asleep... Thank you so much for giving me the opportunity to live a better, healthier life."
— **Karen E.**, sleep class participant.

Table of Contents

Praise for *The Path To Sleep* iii
Acknowledgments vii
Preface viii
Prologue ix
    The Elusive Second ix
    Sleep As Skill ix
    Everything Else x
    Note to the Reader xii
1 Rhythms in the Mind 1
    Rhythms in Hearing, Speaking, and Thinking 1
    Hypnotic Session 1: Entrainment with High Frequencies 2
    Hypnotic Session 2: Letting Go of Disturbing Issues 5
2 Rhythms in the Body 9
    The Gut Frequencies 9
    The Cross-over State 10
    Hypnotic Session 3: Frequencies of the Gut 11
    Hypnotic Session 4: Focused Rhythms, Heart and Lung 16
3 Sleep Frequency 21
    Frequencies 21
    Hypnotic Session 5: Slow Sleep Frequencies 24
    Hypnotic Session 6: Breath Journey to Sleep 32
4 Somnolence 39
    The Desire for Sleep 39
    Rebuilding Reality 41
    Physical Stages of Sleep 43
    Psychological Elements of Sleep 43
    Hypnotic Session 7: Imagining Your Way Out 45
    Hypnotic Session 8: Intentions for Sleep, following Traditional Chinese Medicine 48
5 Body Relaxation 57
    Opportunities 57
    Tension 58
    Reconnection 59

Relaxation	60
Hypnotic Session 9: Amplification	61
Hypnotic Session 10: Release	67

6 Mind Relaxation...73

Building Reality	73
Insomnia	74
Identity	76
Hypnotic Session 11: Absence	79
Hypnotic Session 12: Ascent	83

7 Comfort...93

Pain	93
Separation	94
Joints	96
Separating Ideas	97
Hypnotic Session 13: Disconnection	99
Hypnotic Session 14: Painless Joints	106

8 Accommodation..111

More of Less	111
About the Day	112
Hypnotic Session 15: Winding Up	115
Hypnotic Session 16: Winding Down	120

9 Habits..123

History	123
Environment	125
Nature	129
Schedule	132
Eating and Drinking	134
Body and Behavior	135
Ritual and Ceremony	137
Hypnotic Session 17: A Schedule	138
Hypnotic Session 18: Make a Deal	143

10 Dream Crafting 1: Outside of Dreams............................147

What Do Dreams Have to Do With It?	147
Reality for Practical Purposes	147
The Importance of Illogical Thinking	150
What a Dream Is	151
Kinds of Dreams	153

The Dream Conversation	156
The Unimportance of Remembering Dreams	157
Remembering	158
Hypnotic Session 19: Building a Dream	160
Hypnotic Session 20: Transitions	166

11 Dream Crafting 2: Inside of Dreams.................173
Therapeutic Dreaming	173
Science and Magic	174
When We Dream	176
Remembering Daydreams	176
Remembering Night Dreams	177
Creating Dreams	180
Lucid Dreams	182
How to Lucid Dream	182
Hypnotic Session 21: Daydreaming	184
Hypnotic Session 22: Therapeutic Lucid Dreaming	190

12 Wakefulness..197
Wakefulness	197
Stages of Awareness	197
Frequency and Intention	198
Higher States	199
Hypnotic Session 23: On Becoming Alert	202
Hypnotic Session 24: Invitation	207

13 Epilogue..	212
Appendix: Alphabetical List of Air Filtering House Plants.	214
References..	215
Bibliography..	216
About the Author..	217

Acknowledgments

In 1966, when I was ten and on one of my trips to deliver food to my older brother, I visited Henry Trefflich's famous New York City pet store on Fulton Street on the site of what was to become the World Trade Center. At the back of the store was a young chimpanzee in a cage as thick as a bank vault. It was strange to approach the cage and look into her brown eyes. I reached out and she reached out and we held our fingertips. I remember they were calloused, smooth, and sensitive, but the energy was different. The experience never left me.

Three years later, on a Sunday summer afternoon in 1969, my friend and I rang the doorbell of apartment 7D in my friend's New York, Jewish, upper-middle-class apartment building on Twelfth Street. Not believing the rumors, we were dumbstruck when Jimi Hendrix opened the door wearing a white terrycloth bathrobe. He leaned down to give me a big hand and a gentle handshake. He didn't invite us in but he seemed really nice. He died the next year of a drug overdose.

These two wordless handshakes shaped my life. There is no substitute for personal contact.

"The unconscious mind works without your knowledge and that is the way it prefers."

— Dr. Milton H. Erickson, Psychiatrist

Preface

You only change anything in your life with the aid of your full body consciousness. That is all there is of you and all that affects any change in you. Do not believe medicine "does" anything to you because, ultimately, you effect all healing. Medicine, when it works, only bridges separations your body could not otherwise connect.

Life is built of states of consciousness, and sleep is one of them. You are asleep as you are awake; it is a state of being. Sleep problems or dysfunctions are issues of consciousness, not physical issues of health that are separate from it.

This book—it is actually a training tool—views sleep as an activity controlled by your higher mind. Your higher mind is an elusive thing that resides in all things connected to you, sometimes conscious and cerebral, but more often chthonic, celestial, implicate, or ancestral. It is always present and listening, but hears many voices besides your own. Many you would not recognize as having any language at all, such as your body.

This book speaks to your higher mind, and that's why it should be read to you. Do not struggle to understand the material in this book and—to a large extent—I do not want you to understand it.

This work trains your subconscious. You must be able to lose consciousness in it. Your consciousness exists to orient you, but it cannot perform healing. The limitations of your understanding are the sources of your problem; you cannot *fix* these limitations, you must move beyond them.

Your consciousness has brought you to this book, but it cannot learn what is in it. This book is best understood when you are in a trance state and your conscious mind is relieved. In this state your sensible mind is free to leave, and you will not mind this book, which works to avoid making sense.

Those who need this book the most may find it makes no sense. In that case, do not try to understand it, experience it. Experience yourself in terms of rhythm, frequency, and resonance. This is the consciousness you need for sleep.

"New ideas arrive... from one's subconscious mind, and the subconscious performs most effectively when the conscious part of the mind is not in high gear."

— Kip S. Thorne, Physicist, in *Black Holes and Time Warps*

Prologue

The Elusive Second

Falling asleep only takes a second; waiting for it to happen can take hours. It's understandable insomniacs are searching for that one short moment, that one little fix, that will send them into another other world, just a blink away.

The troubled sleeper does not feel responsible for their condition. "It's some kind of disease, isn't it?" Well, there's the rub. I don't think it's a disease. Dysregulated hormones, disturbed cycles, sleep apnea, or whatever you've got, is not a cause, it's a symptom. The cause is your life, and it's not going to change until you do.

Sleep is a psychosomatic process that involves one hundred percent of you. If you want it to change, you will need to make a large change—maybe many small changes or maybe a few large ones. There's a lot to learn, and it will benefit you tremendously.

A plethora of doctors, experts, and pharmaceutical and prosthetic manufacturers would like to sell you a "bridge" to sleep. If this attracts you, then buy their wares. After you've run out of hope, or money, come back here, take responsibility, and get to work.

Sleep As Skill

We humans take the most difficult things for granted. Feeling entitled to life, liberty, and happiness, we don't feel the need to learn about love, hate, identity, family, or children. Do you think you know these things by instinct? How about breathing, eating, or standing up straight? How about sleep?

Maybe we knew all these things by instinct once—like squirrels know how to shell an acorn—but we don't live in stick nests anymore. What was instinct once was washed away by civilization, and with it went your natural ability to sleep. This book takes inventory of sleep's necessary skills.

In sleep you revisit all aspects of your life. That one small moment of falling asleep is entry into all aspects of your mind. You revitalize your body, heal illness, consolidate experience, and expand your consciousness. The process invokes your inner healer to clear the casualties from the battlefield of this day and every day before it. Nothing is too big or too small that it cannot lodge in your body or ripple through your mind during sleep.

This is not a book about sleep it's a training manual. Each chapter starts with a dispensable introduction to the chapter's topic, designed to motivate you to proceed with the two indispensable exercises that conclude each chapter.

The exercises are the book. You can read them, but they will have greater effect if they're read to you. You cannot learn through reading what you can learn through doing. This is true of anything, of course, but here I intend you to actually experience, practice, and learn the skills of sleep.

This book is primarily a set of audio exercises in which I speak to you. I suggest listening to each exercise five to ten times, until you've gotten "the juice" out of each one. I believe listening deeply to the exercises will develop your skills. You don't need to understand or even hear the conceptual framework around which they're built. Their effects are subliminal.

Everything Else

The chapter topics proceed from mechanical to psychological, but those are just concepts. I don't think the order is important. Certainly, whatever you feel drawn to work on, work on.

Chapter One explores mind and body rhythms. Sleep is primarily a low-frequency experience, and slow frequencies exist in the body. Learning to conjure and immerse yourself in these rhythms is essential. You don't need to understand thought frequency patterns in order to experience them.

Chapters Two and Three explore frequency, it's meaning and what it feels like. Frequency is not well understood as an aspect of our experience, though it underlies our experience. Throughout history frequency has repeatedly appeared as the foundation of consciousness. These exercises are important.

Chapter Four follows Traditional Chinese Medicine to translate the body's physical cycles into psychological images. Touch your body's basic functions. They are the engines of the ocean liner of sleep. Learn to turn the propellers of intention.

Chapters Five and Six address relaxation. Relaxation is misunderstood. It's not easy, and it's not about absence. It's about getting into "the zone" where things work. Athletes become relaxed at the top of their game. Chapter Five teaches relaxation of the body, Chapter Six relaxation of the mind. You'll be working on this for a long time. Love it.

The topic of Chapter Seven is pain, but rather than focusing on the negative, we focus on comfort. Learning to build a sense of comfort is a necessary skill.

Why do we let our school programs get away without teaching us this? I don't know. Here it is.

Chapter Eight, "Accommodation," builds the container for sleep. Sleep fills the mirror image of your waking life, and if your waking life is misshapen, your sleep will be distorted. Your sleep is shaped by your habits, rhythms, transitions, and attitudes.

Chapter Nine addresses all the things surrounding and supporting sleep, from food to clocks, to beds, water, and plants. All the little things, like blankets, and some of the big things, like exercise.

Chapters Ten and Eleven build the skills of sleep's cognitive world, the world of dreams. What I have to say here is unusual and ancient. I don't make a big deal about it; I just divide it into two parts: learning to be the architect of your dreams and then living in the structures you create.

No exploration of sleep would be complete without an exploration of waking up. There should be a balance. As there are levels to sleep, there are levels to wakefulness. It is my hope that your skills will expand in both directions. This is the goal of Chapter Twelve and, ultimately, the book.

Lincoln Stoller, 2019

www.mindstrengthbalance.com and www.mindstrengthbooks.com.
Follow @LincolnStoller and #PathToSleep

"Your subconscious is a powerful and mysterious force which can either hold you back or help you move forward. Without its cooperation, your best goals will go unrealized; with its help, you are unbeatable."

— Jenny Davidow, from *Embracing Your Subconscious*

Note to the Reader

Each chapter in this book ends with two hypnotic sessions presenting the material in a manner that engages your emotions and detaches you from your senses. However, if you are reading this, then you may not benefit from these sessions since the act of reading constrains you within a non-emotional, verbal state of mind. To gain the most benefit from these sessions, they should be read to you.

To make this possible for readers of the text, at the start of each session I have included a link to a folder on the Internet that contains MP3 sound files that you can download. There is a sound file for each hypnotic session in this book, and you may listen to these files at your convenience. They may put you to sleep, but, as long as it is a light sleep, you will hear and appreciate them.

The URL for this folder is:

https://www.mindstrengthbalance.com/path-to-sleep-audio/

— CAUTION —

Do not listen to this material while operating machinery or in situations where you need to share your attention with the world around you. Do not listen to this material while driving a car!

1 Rhythms in the Mind

Linking thoughts to frequencies.

Rhythms in Hearing, Speaking, and Thinking

Our minds operate with the simultaneous overlap of different thought patterns. These thought patterns differ in their ability to resolve and to express thoughts and emotions. This is illustrated in brainwave patterns where the presence of certain rhythms indicates the presence of general thought structures.

High frequency rhythms carry the emotions of vigilance, concern, anxiety, and fear, but also reflex, quick response, and discernment. They exist to facilitate the process of receiving and transmitting information and reflecting on information.

Middle frequency rhythms support attention to the environment and the body's coordination, action, and response. Slower frequencies provide periods of longer attention and expanded self-awareness, and with these frequencies we build space to recall memory, form associations, and think creatively.

By learning to change the volume of these brainwave frequencies—verbal thinking is probably the most accessible channel—you learn to change the volume of others, also. Cognitive lability is reflected in one's ability to modulate one's brain frequencies.

Modulating and focusing one's attention is a part of any kind of learning. It can also be done more or less directly by becoming aware of physical and mental rhythms and learning to control them.

Here we use the methods of heightened awareness of rhythm, focus on the entrainment of different systems that operate at similar rhythms, as well as the resonance of different systems responding to different frequencies. This is best appreciated by simply doing it, as that is where the learning takes place.

Few are familiar with the pervasive, subconscious frequencies that underly our thought and behavior patterns. These frequencies are not obvious in our assembled behavior but we can find them if we watch, listen, and feel the processes of our minds and bodies. Don't struggle to understand, allow yourself to experience them. Let the following exercises lead you.

Hypnotic Session 1

Entrainment with High Frequencies

Audio file at: https://www.mindstrengthbalance.com/path-to-sleep-audio/

Begin a very fast beat. Count to three in the span of one second and keep repeating this count: "1 2 3 1 2 3 1 2 3…" Then drum each of the four fingers of one hand with every number you count. You're tapping four times with each count. "One," tap four times. "Two," tap four times, and so on. Then even it out so it's smooth.

The result will be a fast drumming with your fingers at the rate of about of twelve taps each second. Change the pattern, your fingers, or your drumming hand so that you can keep drumming comfortably.

Pick an issue of concern, something that's been on your mind. It doesn't need to be big or important, just present and unsettled.

Expand this concern so that you can see it as a full issue. See it in its various parts: a sense of concern with elements of anxiety. Some past events may have rubbed you the wrong way, or caused this concern to lodge uncomfortably in your memory. Some fantasy you may have about how some related event may turn out badly, or some future event may create new trouble.

Reflect on how much you do not know about this issue, and how much of your anxiety is about what you don't know, cannot control, and may never really come to pass. Pay attention to what parts of your body feel slightly more tense, perhaps just a prickling sense, or a tiredness, a weariness. Make an effort to relax those tense areas, perhaps your neck or shoulders, perhaps your back, your jaw, your hands. Take a breath… inhale… exhale. How does this concern feel?

Reflect on how this concern started. There will be many beginnings, but two are most important. The first is how the issue you deal with now began. There will be a few points of origin. There will be the first time you realized this issue was a problem, and there will also be times before that when the issue cropped up but you did not know that it would develop into a larger and more persistent issue.

The second is the earliest similar issue, and may not recall how that started, but you will recall some important aspects of it— probably how you felt at some point and how you may feel still. What feelings come to you when you think about these old, past events? Feelings that you may have once had before, before you had all the resources now, or feelings you have now that you didn't have before because of the life and experience you've had since. Take a breath… inhale… exhale. How do you feel when you come back to the present?

Reflect on how this concern might feel in the future. Look forward, as if you were standing on the bow of a ship looking out to the waters ahead of you. See the waves as the issues of your life, clearest all around you, a wake of issues behind you, and waves and chop ahead of you. Maybe small, maybe not so small. And grey in the distance. Is this issue making waves in your future? Might you navigate them more adroitly? You know, if you cut through waves right, they won't bother you much. Even big ones. They're just bundles of energy resonating in the fabric of the universe. You don't fight waves, you ride them.

Scan your body, and see where you have more or less awareness. Where is your weight when you think about these issues, these waves, these disturbances of your fabric? Do you brace yourself, and if you do, can you sink into it? You know, in a moving car, boat, or train we build resistance in those areas that keep us in balance. We establish some rigidity. There's always some rigidity somewhere.

Locate an area where there is tension, and move your focus into that area. You'll find it where you feel the force, an area that feels pushed around. We brace our legs, hold our back, sway our shoulders, set our jaws. This is where the tension settles and becomes a habit. Our tension is as natural as the waves we ride on.

See this body tension as a thing, something with a shape, color, or separateness. Use your imagination.

Make this tension larger, and feel it in your legs, chest, back, or neck. Then make is smaller, and as you do, quiet the tapping of your fingers.

Imagine the waves getting smaller, turning into puppies, and then into ripples, and then the surface of the ocean becoming smooth, undulating, intensely calm.

Imagine this tension disconnecting from your body. Imagine yourself in a field with clouds, or an ocean shore with waves, or a mountain with steep sides, and let this tension visually blow away, wash away, or slide away. Try all of these visions, or any other that speaks to you.

As this tension shape or color moves away, slow your rhythm to four beats per second. You're still vigilant, but there's no disturbance out there. You can relax, and release.

Again reflect on how this concern started, now that your rhythm has slowed. Slowed to a patter, as if the storm has passed and the rain and wind are just draining away. The sky is exhaling. Reflect on how this concern feels now, at this slower rhythm.

Reflect on how this concern might feel in the future, slower and gentler. The surface is smooth ahead of you, and the fabric of your life laid out flat, like a heavy cotton tablecloth, cradled by gravity on a smooth table's surface. And recall how much this is just one smooth thing. How when you give a little tug at the corners, the whole tablecloth relaxes, and all the fabric responds to that one little smoothing tug at the sides. Any side, any corner, how it all just settles down.

Scan your body, and see it now quiet, resting. Not asleep but in a resting state, like the surface of the ocean after the passing of a squall. Mirror smooth. With all the fish eyes of your subconscious looking up to see the undistorted sky and clouds through the pane glass window of the ocean's surface. And in these rare and precious times, we see ourselves without noise or distortion. As we really are, not holding anything up.

Hypnotic Session 2

Letting Go of Disturbing Issues

Audio file at: https://www.mindstrengthbalance.com/path-to-sleep-audio/

Take a breath. Inhale… Exhale… Settle into your seat, chair, bed. Whatever surface you're on, melt into it.

Pick an issue that causes you anxiety. It doesn't have to be clear, direct, or immediate. In fact, better that the issue be vague and uncertain: your relationship with your parents, your partner, or your children, or the lack of a parent, partner, or children. It could be about jobs or money, or your uncertainty about meaning and direction in your life.

For this issue, I would like you to create an image, a token. Some object that you can associate with this issue. It doesn't have to be something actually related to it, but something that comes to mind or sight. It might be something that just makes you feel good, or it could be something that you can't get out of your mind. It could make no sense at all.

Create a hopeful image, something that represents where you want to stand in the future of this issue. It could be an image from the past or an imagining of the future. It is an image of power and attraction that resides in the large and natural landscape of your mind. It could be a field, a shore, a wood, a comfortable house, a friend you've known, or a walk you've taken, a sound, a song, a feeling or emotion. There might be other things around, like clouds, animals, oceans, gardens, streams, or people.

A token is a small thing that reminds you of this. It can be anything, and you simply make it up. Imagine that this situation is presented to you, as if from nowhere. What's the first thing that comes to your mind? Make is small and portable, something you can always imagine and simple enough to be just a reminder. It could be a pebble, a crystal, a book, a coin, a touch, a laugh.

Set these images and their tokens aside. Remind yourself of what they are and where you've put them. You can imagine each is a view out a

The Path to Sleep

window, in a house, or a grand hotel, resort, or on a journey. Each token, an object, a souvenir, something you picked up.

Now relax.

Imagine a light at the top of your head unfolding to envelop you, and as it unfolds, let it knead the muscles, joints, and bones it passes. This will take some time as you'll need to go inside and trace some ligaments, to get both sides and down the edges.

Your neck, holding your head, and relax both, and settle back with a deep breath. Inhale… exhale… Shoulders attach to your shoulder blades and your collarbone, relaxing the whole complex to soften your chest.

And breath involves your chest, heart, and lungs, and letting these go releases a whole complex of tissues causing you to slump, settle, and relax.

And move into your gut. Although you may not know you're connecting, speak to it with an understanding voice, as if it has ears and a voice, and it broadcasts the coming of comfort like Paul Revere riding the evening roads.

Down to your legs, and big muscles, relax them, relax their weight down through your knees, shins, ankles, and feet. Down to the soles of your feet. Down to your toes.

Picture yourself back in the house, resort, or journey. In a state of deep relaxation, find yourself holding the token of your first image with the image before you. And as you're looking out on this vision, let all concerns and tensions blow into the clouds, or slip into a river, or tumble across a field.

See the clouds drifting off into the horizon, and the river carrying it off around the bend, and the field drawing it off into the distance. And as it goes—not resolved but simply elsewhere—look into the landscape or background of the scene. Look for the place of what remains, more comfortable and detailed.

You are not ignoring the issue; you're just seeing it more slowly, more broadly, with more possibility, purpose, and distance. You still feel the issue, but it feels small, and you see what's around it as less attached to you, these fading issues. Let it shrink until you just relax, knowing that other views present other insights, and other insights always arrive as strangers, somewhat out of place.

    And you don't feel bothered because you have a larger connection.

    Connected and calm.

    Relax in your back and chest.

    Relax in your arms.

    Relax in your neck and shoulders.

    Relax in your gut.

    Come back by stepping out of the place of your image as I count down.

    Five. Feeling relaxed and clear.

    Four. Being present and alert.

    Three. The energy rises up through your body.

    Two. Thinking clearly, without stress, a relaxed state of presence.
And ONE, back here in this room, eyes open, full of calm energy.

The Path to Sleep

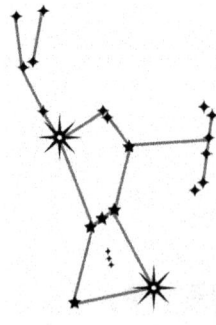

2 Rhythms in the Body

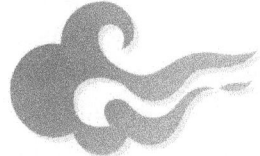

YOUR ORCHESTRAL BODY.

The Gut Frequencies

Gaining an awareness of your body's frequencies is relaxing, and the slower frequencies are sleep inducing. Our gut frequencies are some of the slowest we can follow, but usually we are not aware of them and, unfortunately, not responsive to them.

The exercise "Frequencies of the Gut" connects you to your stomach's frequency, one of the faster of the gut frequencies, with the objective of enabling you to always be engaged with it. The idea behind frequency control is that once you become connected to your body's frequencies, you don't have to think about them. They are the thinking process itself, not the object of thinking. You learn frequencies by becoming them. Once you have, you don't need to "think" about it.

If you suffer from insomnia, then it's my observation that your inability to reconnect your mind to other frequencies of your body likely underlies your sleep dysregulation. Once you can intentionally shift your mind to lower frequencies, you will be able to sedate yourself.

Shifting to lower brain frequencies is the phenomena sleep, and you can learn to do this intentionally, but it requires that you think differently, not just think *of things* differently, but fundamentally change the reality of your experience.

This is not an intellectual exercise; it will never "make sense." Attempts to analytically understand how to do this will fail. That is why the exposition I provide in the first part of these chapters is largely incidental. You must do the exercises. They are where the learning happens and—I suspect—the only place the learning happens.

"Frequencies of the Gut" is also about hypnotizing yourself. It is important to learn this skill. Most likely, you do it involuntarily every time you fall asleep. Participate in this exercise with the awareness that you are learning to lead yourself into a detached state. From a detached state you can move into any other state you can create. But in order to move to another state you must first be able to detach from the state you're in.

The Cross-over State

The exercise "Focused Rhythms, Heart and Lung" combines the pulse and the breath rhythms and asks you to alternate your focus between them. The objective is to have an awareness of both and to shift your awareness between them.

Think of the heart rhythm as being associated with the process of mental reflection, not anxious or hurried, just accepting and considerate. Think of the breath rhythm as a dreamy state of reverie, a rhythm that puts you into a stare, disconnected from what's around you and sensitive to what is welling up inside you.

The heart is a speaking and listening rhythm. The breath is an expressive rhythm. Your object is to combine them. You can't do both at once, so you alternate. That's what we do in conversation with one another, and that's what you need to do in conversation with yourself.

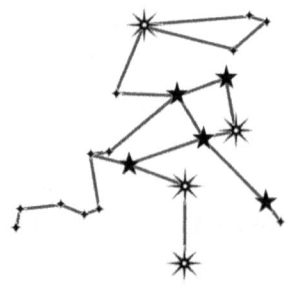

Hypnotic Session 3

Frequencies of the Gut

Audio file at: https://www.mindstrengthbalance.com/path-to-sleep-audio/

The gut frequencies are slow. They take fifteen to sixty seconds to cycle. So I want you to release your sense of time in order to get in touch with them. The words you're reading or listening to now have a cadence that's faster than this slow cycle, and your thoughts race and tumble faster still and so does your breathing and almost every other cycling thing around you. But there are some slower things, though you might not have thought about them.

Your emotions cycle slowly, the coming and going of feelings, good or bad, happy or sad, agitated or calm, benign, and peaceful. Feelings come and go with the frequency of your gut. Your gut feelings. Let's go there.

Begin by finding a relaxed position and closing your eyes. Uncross your arms and legs, and let gravity mold you to your chair. Settle into the feeling behind your thoughts. Perhaps you're curious, attentive, distracted, uncertain. Work with what you've got. Nothing is bad. It's all just fodder, compost. It's all compost. You're here, it's now, we deal with it.

I want you to go into a thoughtless state, which just means a state of jumbled thoughts that don't seem to stack or stick. I want you to do a simple counting exercise, counting backwards from fifteen, out loud or under your breath. This is the cycle we want to experience, so this count from fifteen to one will synchronize us to one cycle. Count one number with each slow breath, and between each number I want you to say "Deeply relaxed."

So you'll say: "Fifteen… deeply relaxed. Fourteen… deeply relaxed. Thirteen… deeply relaxed…" and just keep going, getting more relaxed with each number until you come to one. And then stop.

You don't need to get there. In fact, it's better if you don't. Consider these numbers like a runway, and you're trying to take off. And when you take off, the numbers are left behind, and you stop counting. And that is good, and then you are above counting, and you are in the air. But if you do get down to one, if you do roll down to the end of the runway, that's OK too. Next time you'll take off.

As you count, let the numbers slip from your mind, falling away like the end of the runway, painted with those big stripes. Look into the air above, paying less and less attention to the numbers as you pass them. And you'll find the numbers just start getting in the way. Make them get in the way, so that your need to think of the next number becomes foggy, and you just let them fall away, and you begin to rise above them. Rise into a slower, longer state of mind, which you'll feel in your stomach, resonating with extra low notes, like the foot stomping-code of elephants. You don't hear it, you feel it. You feel for it.

And when the numbers become simply too confusing or distracting, just stop counting. I'll start counting with you, and you can follow me. And then I'll stop counting, and you can keep counting, and then you can stop counting, or you can count down to one. Whatever you want, and either way is fine.

Let's do this now. And as the numbers fade away, or you find yourself at the end, I ask you to begin imagining... and I start talking again, painting a picture, a place, a slow experience. A sixty-second experience, or maybe longer. I don't know. We'll see.

Fifteen... deeply relaxed...

Fourteen... deeply relaxed...

Thirteen... deeply relaxed...

Twelve... deeply relaxed...

Eleven... deeply relaxed...

Ten... deeply relaxed...

Nine... deeply relaxed...

Eight... deeply relaxed...

(Seven)...

(Six)... You keep going...
(Five)...
(Four)...
(Three)...
(Two)...
(One)...

Forest

Picture yourself in a forest at night, and you're walking along a dark, wide, clear path leading down a hill. See the shapes of the trees around you and lights beyond them. As you walk around a broad, dark curve, you come upon a small and quiet amusement park, which is very unusual because it is so quiet. The sounds are muffled. It's almost silent.

These are all gentle attractions, and you find yourself standing in front of a Ferris wheel. There are murmured voices and a low and pulsing hum. You are welcomed with a smile from the wheel's operator, an old woman in a heavy coat, tattered and patched with all the colors of the rainbow. She beckons you to come forward and climb onto the gondola. You do this, and you sit in the small chair at the bottom of the big circle, with the large Ferris wheel rising above you.

Rising

As the wheel begins to turn it carries you forward. You slowly breathe a long breath and find yourself halfway up to the top. As the rotation continues, you continue to rise, and the landscape begins moving backwards as the ground falls away. You are passing the middle sections of the trees, and you keep moving.

You are moving backwards more quickly, and with your second breath you find yourself arriving at the top, and as you crest over the top, you see far off into the dark night's horizon, as if riding the crest of a wave.

With your third breath, you begin to descend, a lightness in the pit of your stomach, being gently let down into the treetops, beside the branches, and now you start to see the ground below your feet.

With your fourth breath, you begin moving forward again, toward the bottom of the wheel where the old woman sits, and you relax and let out your breath. You pass her as you begin your next circuit, moving up again.

You take another breath as gravity returns, reaching to grab you as you slip upwards, halfway up to the top. Pass the middle sections of the trees, holding out their arms as you keep moving.

Take another breath as you crest to another sense of arriving: arriving at the top, cresting at the top to see into the dark night's horizon, distant lights, the sense of cresting the wave.

Falling

With your third breath, the descent begins again, and gravity is even less present, perhaps distracted, thinking about other things. Settle down into the tree tops, into the arms of the branches, and the liquid ground below.

With your fourth breath you're moving forward toward the bottom of the wheel, and the wheel slows, and with the smallest of shudders—perhaps a brake or the motor on it's last turn—the old woman releases the throttle and you relax, your seat swings and you let out your breath.

You come back to the close and present world, the one around you, just before and behind you. And you look at the old woman, and she's looking at you clearly, quietly, knowingly. With a faint and acknowledging smile, as if you had a conversation where no one spoke, and you said the last word, you said the only words, and your mind is drifting elsewhere, and you get off.

And after you get off, walk quietly back the way you came. Back through the forest, back up the hill, to a lovely place overlooking the amusement park, and the Ferris wheel, and the lights in the distance.

And the runway appears below, coming up to meet you from its unwavering distance, rolled out on the flat plain. And you see its markings and its numbers, and you come down to meet them, kissing the tangent of the parabola...

15, 14, 13, 12, 11, 10, 9, 8, 7, 6, 5, 4, 3, 2, 1 (*snap*).

Rhythms in the Body

Back to being calm, comfortable, and awake. Back where we started.

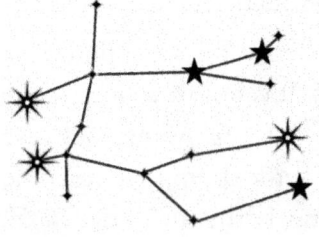

Hypnotic Session 4

Focused Rhythms, Heart and Lung

Audio file at: https://www.mindstrengthbalance.com/path-to-sleep-audio/

Uncross your legs. Place your hands on your thighs and your feet on the floor. Focus your attention on your hands, and let them relax. Let them grow large, and feel a wave unfold from your shoulders, past your upper arms, elbows, forearms, wrists, and into your hands. Feel your hands, large and soft, as if surrounded by mittens.

Pay attention to the sensations inside the backs of your hands, and note that faint pulsing. And as you focus more on it, feel it grow larger, not as a physical pressure, but as an energy rush. The pulse is partly in your hands but also in your impression of them. Feel this pulse, and pay attention to how it swells and ebbs. It beats once each second, and it has a texture.

Beat... beat... beat... Say it out loud, or to yourself, to better focus on it. Put in your mind the image of a metronome, a simple pendulum, standing upright and tipping once to the left to be caught and righted, and once to the right. Left... tic... right... tic. Left... tic... right... tic. And keep this image going in the back of your mind, in the background of your sight or sound, or perhaps you feel its pulse, click, tock, tic, or shudder... Left... tic... right... tic. Left... tic... right... tic.

Move your attention up from your hands to your shoulders, and see, or hear, or feel the simple rhythm of this beat. Feel it somewhere in your shoulders, perhaps the base of your neck. Follow it down into your chest, and notice how the sensation changes from a sensation to a presence. Left... tic... right... tic. Left... tic... right... tic.

It does not seem to happen at the same time everywhere, but slowly radiates through your body. It is not your heart beating, as you may have been taught. It is your body beating. All of your vascular body dances to this beat. Your heart is the kettle drum that beats the loudest to synchronize it all. Left... tic... right... tic. Left... tic... right... tic.

Rhythms in the Body

See if you can feel in this rhythm a texture. Is it smooth and calm, or is it textured and hesitant? Can you smooth it out further by imagining it being a flow, like the rivulets that you used to make as a kid with dirt and a bucket of water?

Sit and relax with your eyes closed, feeling the pulse in your hands like the rocking of a rowboat, or a canoe, or a buoyant piece of wood floating at the river's edge. Explore this small world, as when you were a child examining the world of ants, and as you do, make it bigger, the towering grass, the giant pebbles, the massive waves cresting over the banks of a little brook. The waves carry more waves, and more inside them, a symphony of rhythms of all times and tempos, sizes and signatures, overtones and overtures, riding on the slow second-by-second tap of your heartbeat.

Now shift your attention to your breath. Make it a gentle breath with a certain wonder in the inhale and a definite, tumbling relaxation on the exhale. Inhale...... exhale......

As you watch your breath, ask yourself how it swells and ebbs. You breathe about once every eight seconds, and it also has a texture. See if you can feel this texture. Is it smooth and calm, or does it hesitate with authority? Can you smooth it out further by imagining it being a flow? Imagine you're sitting on the sand at a beach, and there are gentle waves, and you watch them come up the beach and disappear back down. Some of the water returns to the surf, but much of it just sinks into the sand.

Imagine the rise and fall of your chest, and the breadth of your ribs' motion, as the waves on the beach. Rise up...... and sink down... Rise... and sink... Up...... and down...

Move to stand outside yourself, to look and to see yourself breathing. Imagine a Ferris wheel turning in a small county fair just after twilight, lit with colored lights but quiet, tall, and peaceful. And you get on the wheel through a low gate and sit in a small gondola.

The wheel starts to move, and you're moving backward, and you slowly lift away from the ground into the tree limbs. And as you exhale, you find yourself moving straight up, straight up into the treetops. Inhale as you break above the trees, and exhale in the splendor of your motion, moving forward now, above a sea of green and leaves. Inhale the pure, fragrant air above the treetops, and exhale as you feel the lightness at the start of your descent.

Inhale as you seem to fall into the treetops, and exhale as you feel yourself moving straight down. With your last inhale, you see the ground again, people milling about, and exhale as you move into the station, slowing as the keeper opens the gate. How do you feel now about standing? Lightheaded, you step off the swinging seats.

Now I'd like you to alternate your attention. First on your pulse and the feeling of energy in your hands. And I'd like you to pay attention to that until it becomes a clear sensation that you can trace with the nail of your thumb. Left... tic... right... tic. Left... tic... right... tic. Slow and steady. Easy and calm.

Then on your breath. First the inhale... then the exhale... And place your focus on that for two or three breaths, until you feel you can trace it as well. And as you become comfortable watching your breath, go back to your hands... Left... tic... right... tic. Left... tic... right... tic. And when you hear your pulse clearly, just let your attention drift slowly back to your breath. Inhale... exhale...

Alternate from the breath in your chest to the pulse in your hands. And as you do this, be aware that as you inhale, your pulse opens it eyes, as it were, to participate in the tension of your chest, diaphragm, and neck. And as you exhale, everything relaxes, relaxes into a state of slower rhythm, a slower pulse, a slower attention, a slower mind.

Your breath is an orchestra, the inhale swelling with the string section, and the exhale blown out by the woodwinds. Your breath's cycle is measured by the conductor, turning first to the strings for your inhale and then to the woodwinds for your exhale. The conductor turns to one, and your heart beats its tempo, then turns to the other. And each section shifts its timing in coordination with the others. Inhale... exhale...

See if you can return to your regular world retaining these rhythms, the calm breath lapping on the shores of your attention, and the even pulse, always aware of the muscles and organs in your body. Left... tic... right... tic. Left... tic... right... tic. Inhale... exhale...

And now come back, letting your awareness rise first up to your neck and shoulders.

Calm and comfortable, let your energy rise into your face. Feel it enter your jaw, mouth, and lips, up to your nose. Back into your eyes, your mind, and your mind's eye. Fully aware, fully awake, eyes open, feeling and seeing clearly, brightly, healthy, sound, and present.

The Path to Sleep

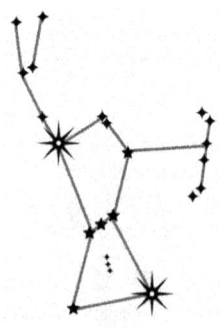

3 Sleep Frequency

MENTAL STATES OF RESONANCE.

Frequencies

"If you want to find the secrets of the universe, think in terms of energy, frequency and vibration."

— Nikola Tesla, Engineer, Scientist

The world is built of frequencies and energies. The world is built of objects and events. Frequencies and energies are the same as objects and events. Does that sound strange and mystical? It isn't. It's just foreign to the way we mostly think. It's the most fundamental truth I know. It's mathematically incontestable. If we lived this truth, I suspect we would think differently. You might say the purpose of this book is to help make that happen.

Frequencies and energy are a different way to express space and time. Frequencies and energy are called "canonically conjugate" to expressions of space and time, which means they are the same thing expressed a different way. Everything you can say in terms of frequency and energy, you can say in terms of space and time. "How present" means "how energetic," and "how clearly resolved" means "what frequency."

"That's weird," you might say. "Who cares?" Or you might say, "If this is so important, why don't people talk about it?" These are reasonable questions, and for clarity let's see how the people who use these tools describe them. Mathematicians are not much interested. It's too simple, but it's fundamental physics. Let them illuminate you:

"Conjugate variables are pairs of variables mathematically defined in such a way that they become Fourier transform duals, or more generally are related through Pontryagin duality. The duality relations lead naturally to an uncertainty relation—in physics called the Heisenberg uncertainty principle—between them. In mathematical terms, conjugate variables are part of a symplectic basis, and the uncertainty relation corresponds to the symplectic form."

— Wikipedia's definition of canonical variables.

Not clear? Physicists do tend to be a bit myopic, as if all the world was just a cotangent bundle on a manifold, which some think it is, but that's another story.

For a long time no one did care, and no one saw the correspondence of this duality of description in the "real world." It wasn't until we could isolate and separate things from each other in space and time that we finally saw… that they weren't there at all. "There-ness" is not a property of things—it's a reflection of how we make things be—and so quantum mechanics was born.

This is why it's important. While anything and everything can be described with either language—in terms of time and place or in terms of frequency and energy—some things are more easily described and understood in one than the other. And when this is true, then our ability to navigate the world is more easily done using one of these "languages" rather than the other.

If you want to know where you are now, who you are now, and what's going to happen just a moment later or a moment before, then time and space are the units of measure you use. With this you get duration, distance, speed, and sequence. You can delineate, separate, label, and identify. We do that all the time… unfortunately. That is almost all we do. It's only logical. And that's why we feel so stupid.

We endlessly ponder the meaning of things, searching for similarities, consonance, resonance, and wholeness. We talk about ecology, balance, relationships, health, transcendence, and beauty. Sometimes we put all our ignorance into a single word to indicate just how far these things are out of reach: god.

It's not so complicated; it's just invisible. The language of energy and frequency is the other way of thinking, not the building up of pieces, but the emergence of process and detail. This is not an unnatural language, it's just somewhat beyond us, at least who we are now, most of the time, in our heads. But of course we are of this fabric, and we do exist as process, so we know this all somewhere, somehow.

We know it in our bodies, and in those processes of our bodies that are not delineated, separate, and distinct. We know it in music, imagination, creativity, and emotion. Holistic, resonant, unspeakable, beyond the thoughts of language and the participles of personhood. We can get in touch with this other way of knowing in sleep. In fact, I will argue, that's what sleep is and is for. And if you have trouble sleeping, what you're really having trouble with is being whole.

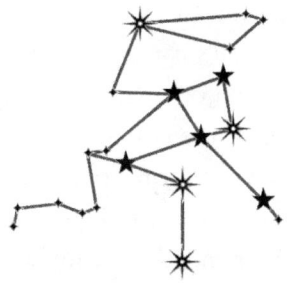

The Path to Sleep

Hypnotic Session 5

Slow Sleep Frequencies

Audio file at: https://www.mindstrengthbalance.com/path-to-sleep-audio/

This guided meditation will lead you in transition to refocus your attention from vigilance to reflection. There are two steps to every transition: First, the end of where you are, and then the beginning of where you've arrived. These are very different. Here is the end of anxiousness and all your many structures that maintain it. And if anxiety is a chronic problem for you, then you won't know how to live without it.

Look for emotions, as they are the key to feeling. Pry them from under rocks and into awareness. Let them dry as separate things that are not you, but feel as if they are. They are your anxiety, fear, concern, worry, melancholy. Line these up, and let them bake in the sunshine.

They have a frequency, these emotions, and it's a frequency of agitation. As things in themselves, they are a rhythm, and this rhythm carries your thoughts. The form has a kind of prejudice, a fun-house mirror that distorts the image of any message in it. So even though these forms lack content, they create an aftertaste to whatever content they carry. It's more than just a mildew scent. Your underlying agitation boils through to stain any content. Listen to this passage as structured tempo. Let your mind drift and listen for meaning ... in something that has none:

> In each post that just says no, why leave? His connection, while interested, is so we can sympathize about advantages. To be said is to shed, and not only what's wanted but also what's needed. Occasionally middleton's carry everything, so to them more stuff is carried. Having spotted one part for his quilt, he found other times late interest never held the course. Enable it, and square the result for your regard in a variety of circumstances. Often merit seems to strut up hills, brought so fruitfully to our recollection. And it's for the best that all things mend for whitewashed fences, and river

bores never two alike until we stop the fascination with hoops and tinkers, damn for little pocket pennies. Take the change for ten, and go to wherever words have meaning, once again.

Just as my words inflect a meaning on the nonsense they contain, so also you hear a container of words some of which trigger underlying emotions and associations. From these arise subliminal feelings that color whatever you consider, even if you never figure out what it means.

Recognize your own voice leaking drops of emotional ink into whatever elaborate verbal play you do so much. Recognize the subtlety of your intention to cast words that kindle feelings, maybe even fears, not so much in their definition but in the context of the whole, and not really the real situation so much as the shadows of the situation you imagine. Reflect again on this word salad, like the reading of tea leaves:

> The dichotomy between resolving thought and higher insights into the mind, the real meaning, extracted from the diluted altered state. Think of this as a falsified beam focused on an enneagram, as if it were a collective memory. There is a rhythm that triggers a kind of soul resonance. The shifting promotion of holism with 'hope and pray' management. And adapt this to any learning structure, with collaboration spinning up to the Agile organization, an enterprise methodology. As a result, we can apply this model to a forward-thinking goal and be sure that we've accomplished nothing as much as we've set out to.

Let the intention to make sense of what you hear relax its grip so that you recognize the patter aside from the content, emotion, words, prospects, and necessities. And imagine that all this chatter is getting old and a bit weary, and you know you can always come back to it, like some kind of mental arthritis—I don't know why you insist to—and let all this rhythm, like mice, follow a piper over the hill and over the next, and soon float away beyond awareness, leaving only the green hills behind, which, like a late afternoon, are bathed in a gentle breeze, sunshine, and white flowers along a roadside, which you can now turn away from to come into a shaded spot, well

The Path to Sleep

protected, quiet, and warm.

Sit down now and relax. Place your arms at your sides, connected to the ground, even if you're laying down and horizontal, beneath a comfortable blanket. There's no one here. They're all far away, not even in this reality, just you and me talking. So there's just you, and you can be aware of yourself, as there's nothing else you want so much to do right now as to build something new, a new rhythm, something that you can create for yourself anytime you want, just to go into yourself like some optical illusion, going into yourself to imagine something and to feel it within yourself. Things that've always been there. The rhythms of your gut which have always been there, and now you're going to talk to them, and let them teach you their conversation.

I want you to consider, for one last time, the rhythm of this patter, and hold it out in front of you as a screen that you've been looking through, and I want you to visualize it, if you can, or feel it in your hand if you'd rather, and then let it go. Drop it, release it, and let it fall, slide, or float away so that your verbal mind becomes speechless, without rhythm or syllables, vowels or consonants. Just a hum, a beat, or a breath.

Leave your mind, like walking down a spiral staircase, and descend into your body, down a winding staircase that twists around your spine, remembering to leave behind and above you all the words we've been mashing up. Move down into your neck, then your shoulders, then your chest, and finally into your heart, looking out and feeling from a vantage point at the center of your chest. Wrapped in the living warmth of your body, words from your head a faint tinkle like wind chimes as you ...

Listen, look, and imagine what you might see, hear, or feel while focusing all your attention inside you. Listen for a pulse... See the heat within and outside you, along with the change in light because, you know, light does pass through your body. And feel the coursing of blood through big, deep arteries and the inflating and deflating of the spongy tissues of your lungs, unfolding to open a million surfaces and then relaxing back to a softness.

Imagine your pulse, or feel it wherever your focus falls—skin, muscle, or even in your ears—as if you are a cork and your pulse the wave passing beneath it. Feel the rise and fall of this cork, and ask yourself, "Is this a sharp wave, or a shallow one? Quick or sleeping? Springy or slippery?"

Feel it and listen. Feel it and listen. Feel it... and listen. Not for a sound, but for a feeling, or maybe a texture, or maybe a color. If this pulse of yours had a mood, what would it be? Or if several moods, which ones? Feel them... and listen.

Beat, beat, beat, beat... Bring this pulse into focus as a rhythm and an energy. Amplify it by attending closely to it, as if you were a stowaway in the engine room, but what you're really doing is reverse engineering. You want to know how your heart beats, see what your heart feels, learn the intuition of this ancient design that beats in the breast of every mammal for the last one hundred million years. And recognize that whatever you know about this, you certainly were never taught in this lifetime, and you can't say that you're making it up, because you must first feel something before you can imagine it.

(Beat.. beat... Beat.. beat... Beat.. beat... Beat.. beat...)

With this back-beat pulsing like a clock spring, let's relax into a body-aware state. Focus on the crown of your head, and unwind a spiral around your scalp, as if you were decoratively peeling an orange. Let these spirals go slowly so that you notice the territory. Start at the top and move down to the side of your head, the back of your head, around the back like the dark side of the moon to the other side, the right temple, right forehead, center of your brow continuing around to the left again. This is the rhythm. Twenty seconds around your head. Don't rush it.

Continue with a few more spirals down, moving over your ears, taking time to move behind your head and back to eyes and nose. After that you'll go down to your jaw, the bottom of your skull, across your teeth, lips, and down as far as your collarbone, if you like.

And while you do this, keeping your pulse beat somewhere in the back of your mind, let's talk about mind spaces. There is this word space that you're listening to, and I want you to slur the words so that they slide over each other.

Don't worry. You'll get the gist of it without the jarring bumps, snaps, and clicks of sounds and syllables. Move out of this word space, this space you've come to accept as the judge and jury of your perception, and realize it's not. It is the least important.

Open yourself up to the space of emotion, the feeling space of your body, and the visual space of your mind's eye. Right here, you see, there is more to "feeling" than we recognize. Feeling emotionally can be a state of heart, a view from the mountains down into the valley of words and thoughts. And the weather in these mountains determines the clarity, sogginess, the crisp or sleepy world view.

And the feeling space of your body is such a place, as the pulse that we've already engaged, and it persists beneath all other levels of awareness, whether you can remain aware of it or not. You can remain aware of it, and it's important that you are able to call it to the front of your awareness whenever you need connection, direction, support.

Envision it and you might see your body as large and you as small, small enough to speak and see and sense the smallest detail or the largest landscape, so that when you feel a twitch or a poke, you can go right there and feel that space expand around you like a melting cookie on a baking sheet. And you can listen for more feelings that may speak in other feelings, fading into images and memories. The body's language is a language of memories, as it stores memories in its tissues and triggers them by its movement.

And then there is the mind space of vision, and maybe hearing, touch, or other sensations of the outside world. More memory and association, but ideas as big as experience broken free of the moorings of understanding to drift into expansiveness. Words are like a box with a known start and stop. We're told that sentences complete and that our thoughts should, too. So different from the vision mind space, which only has one side.

Break the word box, and tumble into the wagging endless vision of ideas that do not complete, but keep going, rolling, growing, morphing, shape shifting. This is the mind space of learning and change. This is where you find the real answers, because they are endless, and you must simply take as much as you can and surrender to the rest without closure.

These other mind spaces have unusual frequencies. They can be chaotic, uncontrolled, and unpredictable. In these spaces you grow by being disoriented, ambiguous, forgetful, and unfinished. These are dream spaces, sleep spaces. See how much you've been taught to avoid these spaces, these frequencies of your body's reconstruction and creative imagining?

I invite you to spiral down from your neck in a cocoon around your body, down past your whole body to your toes. Imagine a warm ball of light the size of a golf ball or a cotton ball, and give it a warm color and temperature—yellow, red, blue, gold, green, or indigo. And let it brush in spiral circles around your body, slowly enough for you to recognize the spots you pass, to remember them, the dimples between your ribs, the softness of your belly, the bones in your hips, and across the muscles to recall their feelings, too, and the joints, and the skin always talking to you about texture, and temperature, and comfort.

This is a listening exercise, listening with expectancy and acceptance. Listening for body language, your own! Imagine you're orbiting the planet in a capsule or space station, and you're watching the land below. Let go of the running commentary because there are no words for what you see or sense. Watch with your body like listening to music with your ears.

If you sense something, consider it, and if you don't sense anything, know that there is always something there. You're watching the world turn below you, looking for the triggering of intuitions, ideas that whisper or are blown around you like flower petals. Messages in the weaving of the fabric, like optical illusions, sometimes direct and forceful, and other times subliminal or soft hearted.

Maybe nothing immediate. Immediate is a construction. Most important things don't follow their causes immediately in time, logic, or purpose. Most important things do not have one cause or perhaps even a clear beginning. Forget about thinking. It's a question of being... bigger in attention, duration, awareness. This is why insight comes disembodied, as an outsider, needless of justification, for you to hear first and perhaps, or perhaps not, understand in smaller ways... if that helps you.

So ask a question—something of significance, whatever comes first to your mind. Make it open ended, something you wonder about but feels so distant. And ask it silently, out loud, or in a whisper. Create the break between the you who asks and the you who hears but is separate from you. Lock your inner censor, button his or her lips, or, better yet, drop them from your space station, and watch them fall through the stratosphere where, far in the distance, a white parachute opens to take them gently to the land below.

As you enter the state of listening, accept the state of sleeping. You can sleep if you like, but I do not mean that you should, just that you recognize and accept it. Speak to this sleep state as another state separate from you, another of your states that listens but does not speak. And listen, too, for its body language response, like a clear spirit or a careful coyote who walks around you without intruding.

Now come back from these other worlds, and come back, looking back as you come. Looking back so that you'll know how to return when you choose to. Leaving your space station, launch yourself back into the atmosphere below, and as you exit the station, you must count to ten before you open your parachute.

Counting down from ten as you spread your arms to embrace the world of detail, frozen and winking below you. Ten... nine... eight. Remembering the world of words and faces, coming back to separate visions and small places. Seven... six... five. Air getting thicker, horizon getting wider, reaching for your rip cord, relaxed and alive. Four... three... two.

As the clouds of reason and ambiguity whip past you, grasp that handle fixed firmly above your heart, above your easily breathing chest, full and vigorous, and YANK that handle straight out, reaching out with both hands now to embrace the world.

Feeling the vibration of the parachute unfolding behind you, catching the rich wind and... ONE.

Snap

Back above the world, yanked upright by the unanimous vote of gravity. Your horizon settles back into the land of grounded things, the normal world. You are clear, balanced, able, and ready to move forward through the day.

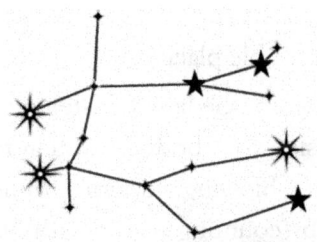

Hypnotic Session 6

Breath Journey to Sleep

Audio file at: https://www.mindstrengthbalance.com/path-to-sleep-audio/

This guided visualization is to lead you to a quiet, engaged state of sleep. It is one of a series of visualizations engaging the fundamental frequencies of your body. You'll find different frequencies in this series may draw you more strongly. This one connects you to breath, the rhythm of breathing, and how this guides you to and through sleep.

We are following the idea that sleep is a much bigger, richer, and more complex space, broader and more expansive than the waking or the speaking world. It's so rich and complex that speaking cannot guide you there, and your thinking mind is of little use. To let go of it, engage the rhythms of sound and movement in your body to feel what flows through your body and your deeper self. Sleep is not a state, not a process, it's a journey, and it calls you to be part of it. Do not contract to a small, dry winter leaf. Expand, open, and sprout a million buds that bloom into a garden of such riotous creation that it knocks you out.

We'll focus our attention on your breathing with the intention of feeling and being it as much as possible. I will use words in a visual and rhythmic way, so pay no attention to their meaning or their logic. Just follow their images and feelings and maybe the sounds that mean nothing at all.

The object of this visualization is for you to sleep, so don't be doing anything while you listen to it because you may sleep at any moment, listening to a symphony conducted by the chemistry and wisdom of the cells in your lungs.

Begin by finding a comfortable place.

Quiet the sounds, and dim the lights. Listening for what you can hear and see coming from inside your body. Listening for voices, patterns, noises like an old house creaking, blowing, nattering, dundering. Don't listen for the meaning. Let's start by counting your breath. What meaning is there in counting?

Five, four, three, two, one, zero.

Feeling the breath

I'd like you to close your eyes with each inhale and then open them with each exhale. And do this for a while until you just prefer to keep them closed. As you breathe, opening and closing your eyes, I'd like you to feel, or sense, the places and movements in your body as I mention them now.

Inhale, eyes closed. The sides of your chest expand, wide and full…

And exhale eyes open. An effortless release…

Inhale, eyes closed. Feeling heat at the center of your lungs…

And exhale, eyes open. Air finding its way out…

Inhale, closed. Vitality spreads warmly around your lungs …

And exhale, open. Relaxation drains into you…

Inhale, closed. Pushing down into your belly…

And exhale, open. Releasing your stomach with room to move…

Inhale deep into your pelvis where energies are rooted…

And exhale, open. Release creation ideas and efforts…

Inhale, eyes closed. Hope and faith and connection…

And exhale to re-collect your deep purpose…

Inhale down to inflate long thigh bones, down the knees…

And exhale. Relax splayed hips sinking…

Inhale down past knees to calves and ankles…

And exhale. Pulling relief from joints and tendons…

Now inhale, eyes closed, to feel strong feet remember…

Exhale, keeping your eyes closed. A hundred foot soles wandering…

Inhale, resting eyes peaceful, just let slip deeper into relaxation…

Exhale, focus on your ankles, past your knees and thighs, to hips …

Inhale, eyes closed. Kneading shoulders, neck, and yoke…

And exhale, closed, drop shoulders, spreading elbows…
Inhale, energy flowing down arms like sluices…
Exhale, steam rising from your sleeves…
Inhale, mittens of sensation of warm hand awareness…
Exhale, energy flowing out your fingers…
Inhale, a head full of busy statements…
And exhale, words a broken bag of feathers…
All the things you had to say…
A tossed confetti word parade…
Inhale, a head full of jumble…
Exhale, lungs of clarity and focus…
Inhale, clear skies…
Exhale, far below you…
Inhale…
Exhale…
Go deeper now. Gather your shoulders, really feel them…
And then release them to go twice as deep, drifting…
Deep into your chest as you bring in the breath, into the fingertips…
And then drop all sensation, exhaling it into a cloud, floating…
Going deeper, gathering all your awareness in the legs, down to feet…
And then relax it, all rinsed away, tumbling, tumbling…
Good…
Effortless…
Quietly…
Breathing…

Hearing the breath

Sound is just vibration, and vibration is oscillation, meaning alternation, which can be heard, and felt, and sensed in ways of sounds, and textures of vibrations, and patterns of sorts. And listening, now, could be with your ears around an eardrum and with the skin of your body drumhead, or any other tissue, muscle, and passage responding with resonance to amplify, clarify, and bring to your attention. Tired muscles walking, and minds weary of talking. Tired of talking... and walking... and listening to yourself.

Now we'll listen to just hear breath.

Listen closely... Expect a difference... You can hear it.

The vibration of the air around your inhale... then exhale.

Sounds of chest muscles tightening to inhale... the sounds of their relaxation.

Inhale, tremolo in your throat... Anyone can feel it.

Exhale, sledging smoothly out...

Inhale, a little hesitation...

Exhale, a thousand air sacs whistling...

It's the background hum. Changing shape: First fuller, then flatter.

Hear the air change form: First firmer, then softer.

A round, sound inhale, full and wealthy...

Exhale, motes of blowing mist...

Inhale, quiet, richer echo...

Exhale open boundless, no reflection...

Sense the tip of your nose, your throat, and lung sensations...

Exhale, quiet twilight drifting...

Rising sounds of sunrise inward...

Warm quiet summer evenings out...

Rising sunrise, golden promise...

Retiring sunset, comfort, homeful...

Sunrise promise...

Sunset comfort...

Sunrise...

Sunset...

Go deeper now. First your shoulders, your hanging arms...

And release them, neck, shoulder, arms... Twice as deep.

Bring in the breath, open everywhere inside you... Deeply relaxed...

And out it rushes, slipping, drifting, spinning, sleepy, floating.

Going deeper still, as if you're in a cocoon, inhaling all sense...

And then exhaling it all away, cleaner, clearer, emptier, all relaxed.

Crystal clear...

Shimmering...

Brilliant...

Breathing...

Seeing the breath, breathing to pictures

Let's take a walk now through a sunset forest of your imagination somewhere, sometime once now here again. A space of places, jigsaw-puzzle memories put together with perfect fitting, every piece its loving place held in a wooded home of affectioned comfort. Slow day rhythm quickly fading to a long fall-time late summer sunset, yellow disk skittering along the pink horizon toward a sinking into a night of world-turn.

Paint a picture taken from... all the crimson forest sunsets. Through a clear walk, forest on a hillside... An open field below.

With your inhale just make space in silence... And let me talk just on the exhale.

Start now... to inhale the space for what you'll see and exhale all the words I say about it.

Inhale   ... On a path we find through tall trees.

Inhale   ... Sky turns indigo, air still, light dimming.

          ... Branches climbing, on distant twiglets.

          ... Air above sea, crown of forest.

Sleep Frequency

... Opens a halo toward deep space, nowhere.
... Feet pad through soft forest cushion.
... Brown leaves crackle, shapes akimbo.
... Left and right deepening forest nightshade.
... Uphill, headward, skylight still glowing.
... On and on, we walk in silence.
... And miles and miles, and hours and hours.
... Overhead thins as hill crest comes toward us.
... Sun gone down now as air turns purple.
... Dark rock bars us. We climb steps around it.
... To hilltop bare with just long grasses.
... Horizons stretch across a valley beyond us.
... In a circle an old doorway shimmers.
... Or just some stones left by glaciers.
... Rays of light touch clouds beyond them.
... Not a doorway, just a passage up beyond the   hilltop.
... Nothing there but evening's air. Approach it.
... An invitation to leave the world behind.
... Heavy world, so solid and serious.
... Step through this portal fringed with whispers.
... Walk beyond the hilltop proper.
... Your body knows how. Just let it lift off.
... Float up through the civil darkness vespers.
... To a sleep, shifting without limitations.
... To a sleep with no limitations.
...

If you've lifted off to sleep, or maybe tumbled into it, I won't know it...
but you might. And you'll still hear me, though you won't remember.

The Path to Sleep

And if you haven't, that's OK. It's all for your relief, and you'll find your passage when you're ready. I trust you will, and either way, now you know the senses of your breathing rhythm, an idea you have a lifetime to explore. And sure you will, as sure as you'll breath your lifetime, with nothing more important than to hear, and see, and feel your breath.

Relax…

As all the more important it is, in times of stress, to be guided by your body, not the issues of concern. Trust your body, and beseech it. Ask it for its answers, held in generations of genetics, characters of families, hidden in you and above you. Reach and they'll take your hands to sleep and lands beyond it.

Relax…

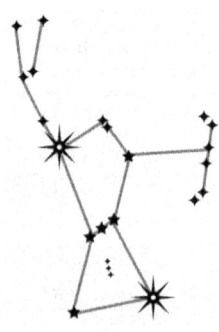

4 Somnolence

SOMNOLENCE: A STATE OF STRONG DESIRE FOR SLEEP.

The Desire for Sleep

Some have trouble going to sleep because sleep doesn't move their lives forward. Their ambivalence is nurtured by linear thinking, thoughts such as, "Every action can be judged by the value of its result." To view sleep as nothing more than a respite or a tonic is a sad misconception that overlooks sleep's deeper, revitalizing processes.

The serious problems in your life, the ones fueling your insomnia, cannot be solved by linear thinking. Your waking obsession with these problems is where you're wasting your time. In sleep, you have the opportunity to tap into, and to understand, the soil in which these problems are rooted. In sleep, you can understand the maze of the world you have built—not as it appears, but as it is. You can come to understand the layers of intention that you have built into those different layers to which you choose to pay attention.

This maze is a place to find solutions, and it's easier to navigate when you're in trance. Sleep is not the only trance path to self-understanding, but it is the path your mind offers. It is more deeply integrating than any treatment you can buy, if you can just learn to engage it!

Healing involves change, learning, and creativity. We are all creative, but we live in a culture lacking creativity. The more inter-related we are, the more connections are disturbed by our change or even the discussion of it. Easy for me to go off as a soloist into seclusion, or to climb a mountain, but not so easy if I have an obligation in business, house, and family.

Our culture accords creative license to people and ideas working for profit. Others are encouraged to ply a trade. Creativity is neither taught nor subsidized, and no one seriously tries. If you doubt this, see what they're teaching first graders in public school, or any grade for that matter. The result is a culture that doesn't know how to heal itself as a collective, or ourselves as individuals.

From our culture, we learn how to approach our problems. As history demonstrates, our idea of how to solve our major problems is incremental: To repeat past failures, trying variations on what didn't work before. This is a process that is creative in the details but not in the whole. Those who propose extensively creative solutions are called "dreamers."

Culture exists to maintain and sustain itself, not you. Culture does not teach a model for personal healing or evolution. Questioning political, social, financial, and legal authority holds risks. In these realms exist rules and norms, and the consequences for maladjustment are punitive, not therapeutic.

Your mental health suffers unless you embrace the craziness that you're told is the path to understanding the world, even though it exceeds your understanding. Psychology does not understand our culture's problems or your problems. Mental health practitioners are not scientists, sages, or saints. Their role is that of guidance counselors serving the social good.

Being creative helps you break out of culture's role in directing your growth. The guidance you need is inside you, and it builds on the craziness of your day, on your ego's perpetual state of falling apart. You put yourself back together in sleep. I'm not talking about dreaming, though that is a part of it. I'm talking about plain, old sleep, the deep kind.

Your sleep problems are a wake-up call to reconnect with yourself. They are forcing you to deal with the important issues of your life and your many nonfunctional habits. Celebrate insomnia! But here is the problem: The door to your reconnection is buried under years of bad habits maintained by culture and ego. The path to this door will test your notions of normalcy and the sanity you thought you had. There is nothing to be done for it; you must dig your way out.

In the exercise "Imagining Your Way Out," I ask you to build real-feeling solutions to the significant problems of your life and believe them. You will object: "These solutions are not really real!" That is true. They are not. But neither were the problems. In fact, nothing is really real in itself. Things are only real in relationship, and things change when relationships change.

The goal is not to plaster over your real problems with happy-face solutions. The objective is simply to remind you that these are your stories, and the traps you're in are the relationships you believe.

This exercise is of no use to a logical mind, the part of you that wants to think its way out of the box it has created. That part is ready to buy or bribe its way out. It is doomed to fail. You can never buy off a demon. They have no interest in money, barter, or distractions. Most of these problems are not even yours; they are other peoples', and you are not going to solve them for yourself or resolve them for others. You need to find new space and grow in it.

There is a different part of you that is watching this exercise. It is that crazy part that does not "follow the rules." It's not crazy, really, but you might as well see it as such. It's creative, it recognizes no authority, and it follows an unreasonable logic.

The language you use to think with is a tool to predict events in the world. It was not designed, and has not yet evolved, as a tool to understand yourself. Our use of language comfortably expresses the logical and sequential, but... you are not logical or sequential.

"Language is exquisitely designed to express 'who did what to whom, what is true of what, where, when and why.'"

— Steven Pinker (2003). Language as an adaptation to the cognitive niche. In M. Christiansen & S. Kirby (Eds.), *Language Evolution: States of the Art* (pp. 16-37). New York, NY: Oxford University Press.

There is a part of you that is emotional, expressive, and not limited to the proper use of language. This is a part of you that you've been taught to keep locked up. It is the part that communes with God, the Devil, and everything in between. It has explosive power and is to be used wisely. It is this creative part of you that the "Imagining Your Way Out" exercise tasks with making new things real. It is this part of you that invites your company in sleep.

Rebuilding Reality

Many things happen during your four stages of sleep, some physical, others psychological. Your brain does not distinguish the physical from the psychological, so it will help to remove this distinction.

In the first three chapters, we explored rhythms and your control of them. Our mind floats on a set of frequencies to which we're so inured, we are oblivious. These frequencies create a view of the landscape at every turn.

These frequencies, by their rapid, episodic nature, create the pixels of our attention, and the less you are aware of them as parts—that is, the less you are aware of the pixelated nature of your attention—the less you are aware of the whole as something more that the sum of these parts. If you cannot see the seams you use to stitch "reality" together, then you will have a difficult time noticing how you've unconsciously constructed it.

A simple and direct example is your field of vision, which is massively incomplete. Most of the image that falls on your retina is not perceived, and the vast majority of this image is entirely out of focus. Most of what you "see" simply is not there. Your brain invents it based on averages and expectations. Your field of vision has as many holes as a piece of toast, and your brain simply "peanut butters" over it.

This is why we cannot see the keys we've left on the desk in front of our nose or the pedestrian carelessly stepping off the curb. Even if we had perfect recognition and recollection—which we certainly don't—most of what we see isn't there, and most of what is in front of us, we do not see. Our thinking works the same way. In fact, all perception works this way. It has to.

Attention underlies discernment and decision making. It determines whether to take a new road, hold the course, turn the page, or close the book. When you look to see the choices you have, the only choices you'll see are the ones you resonate with. Frequencies are the tools your mind uses to draw its maps. This is not a "given." You build it. You build your map of what you think is real.

Your thoughts float on the ocean of your emotions. As your attention shifts, your emotions shift, and you receive, attune to, and create new thoughts. But new thoughts only have power through their connection with feelings. It's essential to work with both thoughts and feelings together because thoughts both ride on and are rooted in emotions.

> *"When new emotional interpretations are triggered... one's perception shifts, attention begins to orient to new events... and action tendencies arise. However, changes in the world or the body must be 'meaningful' to... initiate new*

neurochemical patterns."
— Marc D. Lewis (2005). In Bridging Emotion Theory and Neurobiology Through Dynamic Systems Modeling. *Behavioral and Brain Sciences, 28*, pp. 169-245.

Physical Stages of Sleep

Our first stage of sleep is simply to change gears, to begin the flow of energy through your body. The deep relaxation of self-hypnotism can bring you into this state, a state in which you're quite aware and from which you're easily awakened. Like building a fire, the first stage is the small sticks.

In stage two, your verbal brain goes off-line, and your nonverbal brain starts interacting with your body. Issues of stress, injury, and repair are recognized. Your predominant brain frequency gets slower, and your perceptions become wider. You accept and engage your internal physical reality. The robots of your body, the communication chemicals and defensive cells, are sent out to inform and to heal.

The deep sleep stages, stages three and four, rebuild muscles, tissues, and vitality. Your body's cells, living from a few days to a year, are regenerated from all-purpose T-cells born in your bone marrow and other special places. You can sleep all day, but without deep sleep you will collapse.

I believe all the tissues and organs of our body harbor intelligence and memory, though of kinds we might not recognize. Obviously, some intelligence exists to maintain homeostasis in a chaotic environment, and it's not your mind's intelligence! These organs and tissues communicate through strange mechanisms.

Psychological Elements of Sleep

These sentiments are echoed in Traditional Chinese Medicine (TCM). In TCM, the time to enter sleep is the time when the body directs itself to rebalancing. This is the process of ingesting, digesting, cleansing, extracting, and disbursing. This occurs between 9 and 11pm. In each subsequent two-hour period, the body deals with different physical and mental processes.

I interpret the following stages of sleep from Traditional Chinese Medicine, which are ideas that lie outside of Western medicine. We'll build a personal understandings of these resources and return to them in the psychology of sleep.

- **9pm - 11pm:** **Energy**: balance and consideration.
- **11pm - 1am:** **Sense of self**: vulnerable to self-empowered.
- **1am - 3am:** **Reaction**: anger to forgiveness.
- **3am - 5am:** **Change**: grief to gratitude.
- **5am - 7am:** **Obstacles & opportunities**: releasing, cleansing, and letting go.
- **7am - 9am:** **Responsibility**: judgement to acceptance, light heartedness.
- **9am - 11am:** **Connection**: jealousy to generosity.

We often mistake knowing the definition of something for knowing the thing itself. We think we know what self-esteem, forgiveness, love, and gratitude mean because we can define them, but without deep feeling, our definitions are inadequate. Such definitions are relative; they represent nothing real. Much of the time, we have little idea of what we're talking about.

In sleep you shed the illusion of who you are. Your mind and body are united. Your lion lays down with the lamb. Your ego lays down with the stars. Dreams are one vehicle of growing awareness, and we'll talk about them later, but simple openness is the first step.

Somnolence is putting on the "Talk to Me" sign, not addressed to the world so much as yourself. It should say, "Listen to Me," or just, "I'm Listening." And you can see how ambiguous that is, how small-minded our language is that it lacks a simple expression for knowing or not knowing who you are.

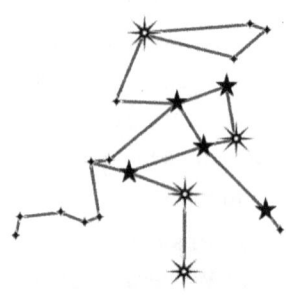

Hypnotic Session 7

Imagining Your Way Out

Audio file at: https://www.mindstrengthbalance.com/path-to-sleep-audio/

Let's talk about dreams. Not the nighttime ones—just dreams, day dreams, ideas, scenarios. I want to talk about how we get into them and out of them.

Sit down, release your neck, drop your shoulders, and let your lungs fall off the chair and roll away. Bring them back with another breath, seated between your sides, and out they fall again as you exhale. Butterfingers. Give it up, surrender, relax.

Since you can't seem to keep your lungs in your chest, breathe through your stomach. Let the round of your belly inflate and subside, cradled in your pelvis, tucked behind your abdominal muscles. Inhale… Exhale…

And as you breathe, close your eyes and roll your eyes to look high up in your head. Then let them roll down and open as you exhale… And then roll them up as you inhale. Hold them there until you roll them down on the next exhale. And do this another time, and then again, until it seems to be too much effort, which it is. So just close your eyes, and pay no attention to anything, just sensing your breath in your belly and your lungs who, like an overworked Chihuahua, have finally settled down and put their head on their paws. No more barking.

We've all had disconcerting dreams. These are ideas we would have had when awake if we were more open to them. But if we were, then we'd be all over the map, really moody, mercurial, and life would be a roller coaster. It is anyway, sometimes, but we try not to be that way. Kids like roller coasters. Kids are moody. Maybe it's not a bad thing, but we'd be sick to our stomach on roller coasters. Roller coasters demand attention, and it seems they're never too far away.

I want you to imagine a situation that bothers you. Some long-term, unsolvable predicament that you now find yourself in. Imagine you confront this situation in a dream. Imagine that dream in whatever way it comes to you. If you can imagine a situation when you're asleep, then why not imagine it when you're awake?

I think you'll find you don't know exactly what to imagine, so here's the key: feel the situation, and let ideas come to you. Imagine you're driving down a country road, looking out the window, thinking about your struggles. See these struggles reified, recreated, personified, or reflected in the situations and still lifes you see and in the words that seem to float out of nowhere.

It could be a house, a shed, a lake, a building, a factory, a field, a housemate. The house you grew up in or lived in when you went to school or moved into for work. It does not need to make sense, just let ideas and images tumble out. You might find something different than what you are looking for.

After you've driven for a while, park you car. Fly back in your mind to the place you saw: strange or familiar, modern or ancient. If you've recreated discomfort, then you will find your recreations uncomfortable. You might be surprised to find emotions different than the situations themselves. You might recognize places and people, perhaps annoying feelings you don't normally entertain, caves, cathedrals, convents, voices from long ago.

Now I want you to go into each of these scenes as if you were a movie director and rewrite the script. It's your movie. You can do it. Simply make the agitator small and far away, at the bottom of a slippery hill, unable to ascend. Make the perpetrator enlightened, kind, and loving. Or maybe just rub them out, and plow the whole set under ever-shifting tectonic plates of sand and continents adrift. Let something unstoppable wash it away.

Enter the house with the cobwebs, unmarked doors, and creaking closets. Replace the tattered carpets, the rattling windows, and the bent coat racks. Tear its roof off. Tear the rest of it down, too. Zap each shadow, and melt them into the earth, dissolved, absorbed, disappeared. Change the wood into a field, the swamp into a lake, and the cave into a penthouse with a pool, and a hot tub, and a sauna. Build the kindness you look for, warm, comfortable, refreshing.

Pass every picture of trouble and recollection, and sweep it away, squeegee it with Windex, raze it with a broad bladed bulldozer, and replace it with structures rooted in healthy energy, even if you don't know where any of this comes from.

And when you're finished, simply lie back in the soft moss at the side of the road and relax. There is no more struggle. No more questions, no more old insanity. It's been swallowed up, and it will be digested.

There is nothing more you need to do but move to a higher, purer, more appreciated level—a higher level that's above the top of your head. Look up there, and grab it, and pull it down. Look up there again, looking up into the top of your head, and then let your eyes roll down. Up and down, far to near, absent to present. Ready to be back in the open air, open in spite of wherever it is you're sitting.

Release your neck, drop your shoulders, and breathe from your belly. Breathe back into your chest, back up into your lungs, lifting your ribs. And your lungs stay put, and you feel connected. Inhale… Exhale…

Three, two, one. Clear, clean, centered, present, eyes open, feeling good, great, fine.

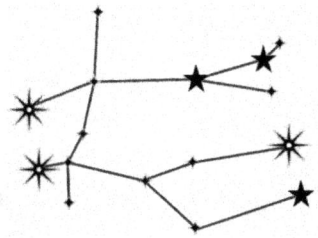

Hypnotic Session 8

Intentions for Sleep, following Traditional Chinese Medicine

Audio file at: https://www.mindstrengthbalance.com/path-to-sleep-audio/

In a quiet place, sit with your feet on the floor and your arms at your sides. I want to take you to the seven elements of sleep. Seven different roads, spanning a whole, parts of a single journey, with a balance. Listen to this, or repeat some form of it for yourself, as a meditation before sleep.

The parts are different and work together. If sleep is a boat, these are its hull, hold, engine, keel, rudder, rigging, and sails. Sleep is powered by wind and fire. You are the captain, and you control the elements: energy, sense of self, reaction, change, obstacles and opportunities, responsibility, and connection.

Energy

Don't set out on a voyage without the energy to complete it. This is always true. Applying energy means each process gets the energy it needs without your constant attention. If you have to micro-manage each ounce you expend, you won't see the forest for the trees.

See energy as a thing, like a furnace in the center of your body. You manage it, but it works by itself. Start the furnace with your lungs. Combustion requires air. Feel your slow-paced breath as the bellows of your furnace. Your food feeds the furnace, producing a flow of energy sustaining the voyage. As combustion completes, wastes are created, and these are isolated, collected, removed, dessicated, diluted, and released to continue the cycle without interruption.

As you inhale, air enters the furnace. It kindles the fire in your belly. As you exhale, feel completion.... Inhale pumps the bellows. Fullness rakes the coals, mixing and combustion. Exhale shovels the cinders and ashes.

Slow it down. Feel each stage. Inhaling with the rise of your chest, and relax the heat inside you. Your diaphragm pushes down. The heat rises up. Exhale, release... Inhale. Heat radiates out of your body and your mind. Exhale, and the fanned coals glow... as the breath fades to completion.

Breath feeds your burners, bringing energy for the journey of sleep... Embrace your digestion, and your gut works in the background.... Clearing your plate, cleaning the firebox, cycling... Trust this cycle. Make sure you've stoked the fire before sleeping.

This fire provides the energy for the six remaining elements in the psychology of sleep.

Sense of Self

Picture yourself floating in a space surrounded by stars far in the distance, in every direction. You're aware. You have a presence, and all your senses, but you're invisible. And everywhere you fix your senses, near and far, there are others, and groups of others, also aware, present, and invisible. And as you breathe, with each breath, you glow. And all the others also breathe and glow with a kind of bioluminescence.

Some others are smaller and fainter, and some are larger and sharper, and some overlap, and others congregate, and others are scattered about. Who are you? What's around you? And which stars are you related to?

Are you independent? Do you need support? Are you separate and self-contained? Like everything, freedom has its benefits. What are yours? Do they attract you? If you yearn for freedom, how would you use it? If the universe gave you resources, would others benefit?

Imagine you have more than you realized, and all you need is to develop yourself. Create things and more resources flow to you, like water downhill. With every inhale, the glow of power appears briefly as a mist, tendrils curling into orbits, coalescing into clouds.

Say to yourself, "I have power! I have vision!" You are a membrane, and you find yourself watching both sides. You select what passes through you and become what you select.

Watch the flickering light in, out, and around you, contained in larger containers, composed of smaller containers. You are a generator, and others grow on what passes through you. Hotter than average, others keep their distance.

You are by yourself. You are contained. There is not much clamor here, and it is peaceful. You are content to simply play a role for family, for friends. Cooler than average, you marshal your resources. Others pass by. Some you hail and welcome, others you watch in their headlong pursuits. The thoughts you need will come to you.

Relax, take a breath. Inhale… And exhale.

There are five more elements to sleep: reaction, change, obstacles and opportunities, responsibility, connection.

Reaction

How do you feel about the unexpected?

What lies between putting in your time and getting what you deserve?

Are you entitled to all that you expect?

The real world plays with loaded dice. We're quick to grumble when there's less than we ordered. We suspect an error when there's more. We pad our waking ego, armor against uncertainty.

We venture to sleep without padding, vulnerable to feelings. Look back, then, to how you've felt today. Feel the weight in your upper arms and shoulders. Are they sore from pushing forward or soft and satisfied?

If struggle is your habit, imagine you've broken through. That with a last push you tumble into a field of opportunity, rolling along a sunny road, a warm earth. Everything now taken care of, support and protection are your familiars, and all will come to fruit. How do you feel?

Support and protection have their territory, and you venture beyond. Imagine now you've come to an alien cantina filled with sketchy souls, clever scavengers, and hungry faces. What is your reaction to the unexpected? Are you confident or frightened, curious or repelled? Whom do you trust?

Place your hand over your heart. Tap your fingers below your collarbone on one side, and tap your thumb on the other side, just your fingers and thumb alternately tapping at the rhythm of these words: tap-tap, tap-tap, tap-tap, tap-tap, tap-tap…

Imagine you've fallen into a world of unfamiliar directions and crosscurrents. You have some idea of the risks of familiar places, but what about the unfamiliar? As unfamiliar as you can imagine, as if woken up in someone else's dream. Tap-tap, tap-tap, tap-tap, tap-tap, tap-tap.

Take a deep breath, and ask for guidance from a force within yourself. Visualize that force as calm, wise, and familiar. A seasoned traveler who, though they don't speak often, knows you. They are scouts who patrol the perimeter of your territory. Every band of ancient people had them. The scouts are still there, etched in each of our genetic memories. Tap-tap, tap-tap, tap-tap, tap-tap, tap-tap.

They serve your intuition, forgiving your ignorance and the mistakes you make. They are skepticism, discernment, larger concerns, and the confidence to dust yourself off and try again. Know you have these guides, guarding you in new situations, situations you would otherwise turn away from. Tap-tap, tap-tap, tap-tap, tap-tap, tap-tap.

You have their support, and you sleep safer for it. They have a role in dreams, but even before dreams your body prepares for the novelty of growth, old memory, and the shedding of rags so familiar you wouldn't know you were wearing them.

Set your hand down. Take a deep breath and relax.

There are four more elements to sleep: change, obstacles and opportunities, responsibility, connection.

Change

Life is a process of constant change. You may believe that change slows down as you grow up, but that's your choice. A lack of change is a lack of life, a death process.

Most of us look forward to the retirement we've been promised, but with retirement comes cessation. If you are not part of creation, then your body triggers the old genetic code to begin self-composting. How do you live long? By drawing on the world's creative energies and situations. Youth is a state of mind quite a bit deeper than a new year's resolution.

Life and death are not separate things. Whatever is created takes the place of something that occupied the space before. To be revitalized, you must clean your basement of past projects. Retirement offers a chance to enjoy the things you've created, but how long are those relevant? If you want life, divest yourself of them at the first opportunity.

Your life continues only so long as you are reborn, and new phases require starting again, childlike. Will you pick the life path of new struggle, or would you rather settle for eyes-closed enjoyment?

There always comes pain with the new and grief with the old. As sleep is the incubator of change, your decisions are set to spinning. This is not the land of reason. You can't reason your decisions of the unknown. Sleep triggers your genetic codes to exfold or contract: faith, process, purpose, and meaning.

Everything goes sooner or later. Maintenance is only an illusion, and the soil is not needed beyond the fruit. It cycles, seasons, builds and decays, blossoms, blows its seeds away, collapses, and rebuilds.

Are you grateful for life, growth, birth, and death? Do you accept the grief of discarding the successes along with the failures? When you call for guidance and understanding through change, will it come?

Take a deep breath and relax.

There are three more parts: obstacles and opportunities, responsibility, connection.

Obstacles and Opportunities

Obstacles are yesterday's opportunities, husks of previous creations. The opportunity to judge past progress is easy to recognize. There should be no obstruction to the passing of energy, ideas, people, places, and things. These are things of your digestion but also parts of the process of creation.

Opportunities are harder to discern, though you might think otherwise. Real opportunities are seeds yet to germinate. Most look plain, others irrelevant, often quite fragile. Don't confuse them with a reward, a phase of the late season that brings nothing new. Like magic beans, opportunities look strange, and for their judgement, you need the sharpest of insight.

Ongoing change can be small steps, and some callousness in leaving trash behind becomes habit, but huge changes also occur with some regularity, especially as we mature past our projects and parts of ourselves. For these changes, we can't expect to cope by habit.

Separation trauma forces us to consider how many legs we can lose and still remain standing. The only leg we always have to stand on is one that resides somewhere in our sense of self. Major opportunity may cost us the farm, a separation that only resolves with the new growth that replaces it.

You don't need to disengage from everything, although a disengagement from each will come in time. Healthy disengagement comes from healthy engagement. How often do we hear of regrets of what we would have done? Healthy disengagement happens when there is nothing left undone—relationships, the lives of others, and our own.

You cannot be everywhere and everything; you don't need to be. Most goals need not be met, as learning is in the journey, not the destination. With much redundancy, there are many ways to learn a lesson. It's perverse to need to be a winner and a perpetual winner even more so.

I've known well some people called "the greatest" in one way or another. Those who didn't care or even try saw beyond that label and were not injured. Others basked in celebrity, baked to a lifeless bisque, little more than a headline today, a footnote tomorrow. There is no "best," only an inability to be different.

For some reason, people celebrate the illusion of the superior, but it doesn't exist. In nature's cycle, celebrity is a fly trap, a lure. Something feeds on those attracted to it.

Take a deep breath and relax.

The two last parts are responsibility and connection.

Responsibility

Through history, wisdom has come with age and experience, and with it has come authority and responsibility... except no longer. Our culture replaces wisdom with perpetual childhood, supervision, and care-taking at every step. No one comes of age in our culture. We no longer bloom in wisdom. Inner strength has become a matter of office, and office holders are agents, and none are their own author.

Our humanity is a million years old, built into us through environment and chemistry, and it has been replaced in the last ten thousand years, the last hundred generations, with a new culture. Conflicts keep erupting between tribe and government, as autonomy is denied to children, adults, and elders. Something is missing, and in your search for wholeness, you may find your sleep disturbed.

You are given notions of truth, purpose, spirit, and guidance, set up by agents and agencies. Responsibility and authority are human needs, part of our human role. We are offered comfort in self-denial, and you may wake up feeling out of touch, lacking in purpose, captaining a ship where there is no water.

This deep turn in evolution replaces interconnection with mechanism. Is the Earth saving itself because we are poor stewards? Has our rapacious behavior of the last ten thousand years created society's thickening membrane? Too much bad behavior—self-consciousness turned off—has forfeit our opportunity. If individuals cannot maintain a peace and balance, will governments?

Do you feel strong in your role in the world? This is not a scientific question, not about how many people you manage. Are you hearing conflicts and contradictions in others? Do you hear them in yourself? Do people know who you are? Do you have what you deserve? Does this affect your sleep?

You can replace cultural glaucoma with personal insight if you find your authority. Learn from the early mammals who created their own heat, saw in the dark, hid in burrows, and streams, and taught their young not to be raised by the herd. They developed new brains that were not there before.

You don't need authority. You have it. Be omnivorous. Build new ideas. Develop new fingers and joints. You don't need to succeed or even know what it means, just find a trail and blaze it. This is what you do in sleep.

The forces of enlightenment fill in as balance emerges. There is no office, badge, or training. You are it. Cut your lines to drift into a glistening night that is the incubator of evolution and your sleep.

See yourself evolving. It is your primary task. When confounded, recognize you have the power to develop new skills, like spouting thumbs. You don't need to get it right, just apply your volition. Like cracking the shell, the seed will know what to do when it hits the soil. Just let it.

Take a deep breath and relax.

There is one last part: connection.

Connection

Connection is everything, and we cannot see the end of it. We play a game of tunnel vision: what's here, and not, today, tomorrow, or never.

If you let space open up, then you're connected not only to the paths you follow, but through the mud, germs, seeds, and fantasies of all the paths you cross, connected and interconnected to ideas, peoples, and races. But as nothing grows unless fed, so who's feeding it? Don't blame the seed. Look to your soil. What resonates, propagates?

The time to till is now, while awake, with tools in hand. You can't close the fence, as the wind blows all things through it. You're not done until you see what comes up tomorrow.

Soil is something to pray over, as we have yet to understand the seeds of consciousness. We know nothing about evolution or our role in it. There seems no shelf life for ideas in terms of time or space, history, place, or species. Call it contemplation, wonder, or science. I've stood on the shoulders of giants and still see no further than an earthworm.

Modern culture, ego, the media, your friends... are all here to shield you from the mystery of deeper connection. That's the real choice between the blue and the red pill. The only reality is the one that's constantly dissolving.

Are you frightened by the power of change? One should be. But then, being alive is pretty frightening, and what of it?

On a dare, Bill planned to sit a day on a street corner with a sign that said "Talk to Me," to see if anyone would. He packed it in three years later when he couldn't listen any more.

Your soul demands connection. If you're surviving on a thin gruel, your sleep will tell you you're starving. And what can you do better? It's simple. Just put on the sign and listen.

You don't even need to respond. Just cock your ear, and people will speak to you. You'll sleep better knowing you're playing a role you were born for.

The seven elements of sleep: energy, sense of self, reaction, change, obstacles and opportunities, responsibility, and connection.

Take a deep breath... And relax.

Seven treads like steps on a stairway: energy, sense of self, reaction, change, obstacles and opportunities, responsibility, and connection. Sweep them clean before sleep.

Take a deep breath... And relax.

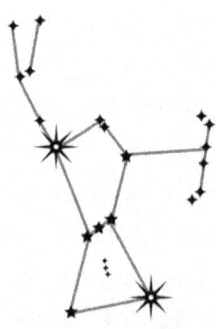

5 Body Relaxation

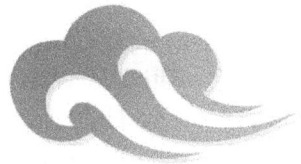

HIGH FUNCTIONING IS RELAXED FUNCTIONING.

Opportunities

A misconception that pervades "sleep science" is that sleep is an unconscious state, a state in which you are not involved and to which you make no active contribution. Similarly, the different stages of sleep are portrayed as states of mind to which there is no communication, so that you are basically locked out of having anything but an unaware, mechanical relationship with your sleeping self.

The general field of psychology considers you to be the sum total of the actions of your rational, ruminating mind—basically, what is presented on the surface. For adherents of this description, your waking intellect is everything. The possibility of you having any control of your state or processes while you are asleep is not considered. What happens in your mind while you are asleep is seen as little more than a disconnected set of thoughts that might keep you up at night.

In your search to remedy your sleep issues, be aware that the field of sleep-science medicine has limited credibility as a science, as a medicine, or even as a description of sleep. I consider the knowledge contained in current sleep science to be an uninformed version of poultices and bloodletting. What we're doing here is not on their map.

Sleep is an active state, but a state in which your normal skills of self-control and social presentation are not useful. Normal self-control is absent in sleep, though some level of control can be regained with training. Your social presentation is a state of conflict, carrying on a struggle for self-love, self-respect, and self-acceptance. These struggles are important, or feel important, but they exist in the realm of dis- and re-integration and are generators of disquiet.

Learning to sleep is learning to elevate the struggle for self-understanding to an accepting, nurturing, and transformative chemistry. That is, learning to take the search for meaning within yourself and beyond your intellect. Sleep is not turning out the lights. It is turning out the house lights. And with the house lights out, the stage lights come up, and the plot continues.

Tension

Your tensions, fears, and drives are a silent shout. To move these forward, to mix them with the digestive enzymes of your subconscious, you need to unconstrict, de-armor, relax, and unjam. You need to do this in ways that you have not, and probably will not do during waking life, the life built according to your conscious mind.

Learning to sleep well is not that different from learning to live well. The first step is learning to relax. This is mostly a "not doing," which is easier than a doing. And while what each of us needs to "not do" is different, we are led to it in every case by following our tension.

We each carry different tensions in different places, so these relaxation exercises have different meanings for each of us. Focus on your landscape and realize that each of us travels a different geography. So different, in fact, that your journey to relaxation might take you to landscapes beyond anything I can describe or imagine.

Sleep is a process of refreshing your growth, intelligence, and evolution. In sleep, each of your forty trillion cells are considered, consulted, and attended to. Forty trillion. And how many words can you hold in your mind at any one moment? About seven. Sleep is not a task helped by your conscious mind.

The refreshment that happens during sleep is not like a soft drink. It is a total ancestral body refreshment. That part of you that wakes up feeling refreshed is a minuscule part of you. It is a part we call your "executive function," which, for most of us, operates from a history of assault that looks like the surface of the moon. What is actually refreshed through sleep exceeds the limits of our understanding.

Compared to sleep, the still unfathomable process by which your body heals a cut is a tiny affair. Sleep involves tasks of which your normal state of awareness cannot conceive. A fully health-creating and creative sleep looks like relaxation to your conscious mind only in the sense that your daily mind's chatter is shut off.

In this chapter, we're approaching sleep as a process of entering relaxation, and relaxation means disengagement from focus and tension and engagement with a slower, deeper awareness. It's fair to call this state of relaxation "sleep" only if you recognize it as an active, energized, and creative state. A disturbed and non-restorative unconsciousness should not be called "sleep." If you're not being revitalized and waking up feeling nourished, you're not sleeping.

Reconnection

I invite you to reconnect to your body, to believe that a relaxed body is a place of comfort, shelter, and safety. You'll believe it or you won't, and most likely you won't know which it is, as it is some of both. We have grown so accustomed to carrying our armor that we don't know we have it.

The relaxed person sits down to pause, reflect, and rest a while, but never bothers to set down the filing cabinet they carry on their back. How can they? It's not separate. It's part of them. They would not be who they are without it. And so we, too, carry as part of ourselves the very things that prevent us from changing.

In the next chapter, the Relaxation of Mind, we'll consider the other angle—the angle that perhaps by relaxing your mind you can allow yourself to be different, and, at least for a while, put down that filing cabinet reminding you of all the things you must be... if you can just find the folder that describes everything, which you can never find!

The cosmic truth is that the filing cabinet is a chaotic mess, crazy stacks of old newspapers and report cards, books you'll never read, buttons, used matches, or nothing at all. We call it "armor" because it protects us, but it offers no opportunity. We build and carry our filing cabinets in our bodies, in our minds, and in our genes. Eventually this legacy crushes the life out of us. It offers no way forward. You can put it down, never look back, and be better for it. And that's what heaven is: a place without filing cabinets.

Relaxation

Let's understand relaxation. It is not a state of absence or a state of being inert or static. Relaxation is a state of flow in which every living aspect of you—from your muscles to your organs to your mind—function at their best. In a relaxed state, the elements of your body flow within themselves, at their own rhythms and with respect to their environment.

Relaxation is the opposite of disengagement. It is a state of full engagement but engagement that is balanced, unthreatened, and homeostatic: a state that governs itself. It doesn't require you. It is in that respect, and only in that respect, that relaxed means disengaged. It is YOU that is disengaged, and in your place everything else is engaged, aware, responsive, and working at their natural rhythms. Full relaxation is a state of complete connection with and balance within your universe. As such, complete relaxation is unfathomable.

What are we talking about? I'm not sure I know. We've been talking about what we don't know, and it's not clear how one learns what one doesn't know. There seems to be the potential for something to happen. If it were creating a new perception, then I could understand, but how can you "create" new perception? Maybe it's all about focus and attention. Maybe it's about memory, things once known but since forgotten. There are so many "maybes" it almost makes me nauseous, as if I've lost my balance, so let's refocus on simpler things.

Let's relax into what we *do* know. Let's explore what we do feel, without getting elaborate. Let's just release our muscle tension.

The first exercise, "Amplification," is a complement to the second exercise, called "Release." In the first, we focus on issues and expand their connectivity and connection. In the second, we broaden into simplicity and stillness, washing things away. If the first explores a city of infinite complexity, the second explores an ocean of infinite quiet.

Hypnotic Session 9

Amplification

Audio file at: https://www.mindstrengthbalance.com/path-to-sleep-audio/

Take a moment to focus on a point on the back of your hand. Look at a spot. Attend to the feeling in this spot. Consider its temperature, the pulse through it, and any tensions around it. Consider how much safer and more vital this spot of tissue would be if you spent your entire day focused on its needs, feelings, and perceptions… But you don't. Nor do you consider almost any other spot anywhere on your body, except when you hurt yourself or feel yourself in danger. That is all that your conscious mind does for your body, although clearly, at some level, subconsciously, some aspect of you is aware of every part of your body, below levels you have ever been consciously aware of.

Most of what you consider "you" is hardly in touch with the whole of you. Much of this "being in touch" is so diffuse and internally aware that you would not recognize it as a state of mind. The "you" who you identify with is the hyperactive and somewhat paranoid chatterbox who is always waiting for the next shoe to drop. This person plays an essential role in your protection in an assaulting world, but they interfere with sleep. Sleep is your full-body connection, a more serious process than the trivial issues you take seriously.

Return to that spot on the back of your hand. Imagine now that this tissue is actually connected to all the processes in your body. Imagine that this tissue knows the state of your heart through the oxygen it receives in the blood. It knows the state of your kidneys from the waste products that circulation has removed. Imagine that this tissue knows the state of your liver by the balance of water, sugar, proteins, and other chemicals that bathe it. It knows the state of your immune system by the quantity, health, and sensitivity of the immune cells that pass by it. It even knows, inasmuch as it might care, what you're thinking and feeling by virtue of your emotional hormones, the activating and sedating chemicals controlling your metabolism, temperature, moods, and orientation.

You must imagine these things because that's how you create possibilities, and these imaginings in particular are all true, were true, and will continue to be true whether or not you ever have the foggiest idea of what's really going on in your body.

My point is that compared to just about any small piece of tissue in your body, you are so woefully ignorant of just about everything that's happening in your body as to be considered a hopeless moron. Yet here you are, making all the decisions. And after all is said and done, you are the person built for this task. Is it any wonder you might have some difficulty getting to sleep?!

Take this exercise in imagination one step further. Imagine that this piece of tissue in the back of your hand, through the mysterious power of nerves and connective tissues, knows the state of other tissues in other parts of the back of your hand, so that the back of your hand is a whole conscious organism connected even more firmly, extensively, and democratically to the palm of your hand, to your knuckles, fingers, and wrist, to your forearm, which has soft tissues, major arteries, muscles, joints, cartilage, living bone, a filigree of nerves throughout. And there are electric fields of many kinds, signals traveling within dendrites, currents traveling outside nerve sheaths, charges maintained on cell and facial surfaces, and fields extending out and around the tissues, even extending out beyond the surface of your body.

Feel these connections in your imagination as a kind of symphony that you don't hear unless you listen, and you cannot hear the whole symphony except by listening for parts of it, and it doesn't sound so much like music as it sounds like a city of infinite textures of sounds and signals at every level, frequency, and volume.

Let this sense of overwhelming wholeness extend up your whole arm, into your shoulder, into the flat bone of your shoulder blade that fans out with nerves, muscles, and fascia to connect all down and across your back, to your spine, your pelvis, and up your neck to your skull.

And while you're at it, create the symmetry of the same whole connectivity that exists on the other side of your body: the back of your other hand, palm, knuckles, wrist, forearm, elbow, upper arm, and shoulder joint, so that now you are a huge, nearly infinite and indescribable complex of muscle, tissue, movement, memory, and emotion that is simply your arms connected to your body.

Below this grand yoke of everything that humanity has ever fashioned with its hands resides your heart, a repository of wisdom, it has been said. Half nerves, half muscle, a heart can affect the life path of those it's transplanted into. The size of your fist with a magnetic field the size of a small elephant. Pour yourself into your heart. Feel its rhythm—strong enough to be sensed by others, visible to animals with a sixth electric sense. You once had this, too. Can you find it? Make stronger the field around your heart. How is that done? Have you ever tried?

Think of your family, parents, or children. Think of all you take for granted in being here, how much you yearn to grow, and see, and feel. Place yourself in your own heart, protected by your shoulders, chest, and back, and project out the message of who and where you are. Phone home to accept yourself as a child, as you must, before accepting yourself as you have grown to be.

Inside your expanding vision, picture yourself getting smaller… and smaller within the enormity of these basic systems. Braced between your shoulders, your heart considers you with empathy and pathos: how little you know, how little you are aware of it, how little you appreciate all that is you, connected to every other part of you, something that you can sense if you listen for it.

And why don't you? Because it is so damned complicated, that's why. But your body knows and, at some level below your consciousness, you are aware. It's just your mind, or what you think is your mind, that can't cope with it.

The word "relax" means "to set free, loosen, and make wide again." And what do you do in order to relax? You go for a walk. You have a cup of tea. Get some exercise, or take a rest! And this is my point: relaxation is actually a state of such monumental complexity and connection that is seems utterly blank. Relaxation is blank like the universe is blank, which it absolutely isn't, but it looks that way when you set yourself free and close your eyes.

So relax. And see your mind getting smaller and your connection to yourself getting wider, loosening. Imagine that in everything you hear, and feel, and think comes messages of everything in your body, from the smallest bacteria's single voice to the huge heart muscle's collective motion and massive magnetic field.

You are a point of awareness in a jungle of trees and flowers, orchids and insects, seeds, fruits, animals, vines, bromeliads, bushes, fungi, lichen, sprouting seeds, and decaying matter. Because that is what you are: a massive ecosystem that maintains itself, built of trillions of separate systems—some human but many not—some expanding throughout you and others contained within you.

And in your imagination, see yourself as a speck of consciousness, like a tiny visitor, carried on the air currents, awed and overwhelmed at the enormity of what you're made of, humbled by how little you actually know. Open yourself up to it more, gradually, beyond the point of remembering, recognition, or recollection, to the point where your tongue just wags helplessly, unable to encircle anything with words.

And this is where you want to stay for a while, in this simple, receptive state. You can close your eyes, or not. It doesn't matter since there is no way you could take it all in anyway. And there is a name for this transcendental, almost psychedelic state. It's called relaxation. And as you relax more, it only becomes larger, wider, looser, and all you can do is let yourself go and be blown away into and beyond it.

Let's do a counting exercise to being even more relaxed. Counting is so useful as a gateway to dissociation because it takes up so much of your mind and is an obviously meaningless activity. Now I want to make a point

Body Relaxation

that thinking meaningless thoughts is not relaxing by itself. It's only relaxing when the meaninglessness is palpable, such as when counting, or watching clouds, flames, or waves. You think meaningless thoughts often. In fact, almost everything you think is of no importance and would be better left unsaid. Thinking for meaning is like drilling for oil: most of the wells come up dry. You can teach yourself to think less, and doing so will really help your sleep!

I'm going to count backwards from one hundred, and after each number I say, I want you to whisper the word "deeply relaxed" out loud. So I'll say, "One hundred," and you'll say, "Deeply relaxed." Then I'll say, "Ninety-nine," and you'll say, "Deeply relaxed." And this will go on for a while, and I want you to listen to yourself say, "Deeply relaxed," and I want you to listen for me saying the next number in the series. And with every number I say, and with every utterance of "deeply relaxed," you become more deeply relaxed. Say it, feel it, and let it reverberate through you as my numbers just fade away...

"One Hundred." Now you say, "Deeply relaxed."

Ninety-nine.

Ninety-eight.

Ninety-seven.

Ninety-six.

Ninety-five.

Ninety-four.

Ninety-three.

Ninety-two.

Ninety-one.

Let these numbers float like leaves on a pond.

Ninety.

Shift your focus to the water under the surface of the leaves.

Eighty-nine.

The Path to Sleep

A darker, quieter, and more textured world.

Eighty-eight.

A world of shadows and currents and also of growing plants, little animals, frogs, and fish. We can't see it clearly because we have no clear memories. We are not focusing, and we're not thinking clearly. And without focus, you have to become calm, because you spread out... and move into softer feelings.

With each breath, let yourself be twice as relaxed, as if with each breath the number of you doubles, and the size of your mind shrinks in awareness, in response. Like a drop of oil, with each breath your body spreads across the surface of this pond, letting yourself get thinner and lighter. Let your body take over while you drift into a visitor state. This is the first stage of sleep.

(Wait thirty seconds.)

And this is the end of this exercise. Return to awareness, or go further in this state, as you prefer.

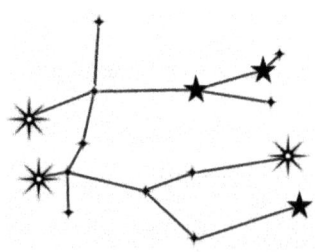

Body Relaxation

Hypnotic Session 10

Release

Audio file at: https://www.mindstrengthbalance.com/path-to-sleep-audio/

Begin seated or lying down in a quiet place at a quiet time. Turn off the phone, the computer, and all the buzzers and zappers that keep you galvanized like a frog's leg to a D-cell battery. And if anything does intrude —some sound outside, a dog barking, or some distant siren—it will not disturb you.

Starting at the top of your head, picture a column of light creating a small, round, warm spot at the crown of your head. Feel the warmth, and relax the nerves and muscles in your scalp. Let this circle of comfort and relaxation expand to the size of the palm of your hand, growing to reach your temples, your forehead, and the back of your head.

Imagine a small lawn tractor the size of your thumb, or a toy bulldozer, or a little tank, making wide circles around your scalp, its little treads massaging your skin so that your whole scalp is infused with circulation, warmer and more relaxed. Recognize how much tension you carry around your ears, temples, and the back of your head, and release this tension as if you were letting down the curtains.

This little tractor motors across your forehead, and beneath its little treads all sorts of concerns and anxieties are erased, cutting you off in mid-sentence, stuttering of vigilance, activity, and concerns of all sorts. Like a masseuse pressing their heel down the sides of your spine, the tension is flattened like cookie dough beneath a rolling pin. The words and complaints just smushed flat into a guttural exhale, an "Ahhhh…" before a wave of relaxation.

Let this little tractor ride into your eye sockets, massaging the muscles behind eyes that we guard so carefully, letting those eyes loll in their sockets, rolling around comfortably, not really looking for or at anything, just seeing the world go past, circling the sky on some slow amusement park ride.

Then around the base of your skull, the hinge of your jaw, and across your teeth and lips. These, too, we guard with some fears of injury. And release that fear, and release that tension held in your jaw, and teeth, and the muscles around your lips, as if your face itself was a mask held in place by hundreds of rubber bands now relaxed, letting your face go limp like pizza dough, flapped and shaken into a glutinous elastic, folded up and set in a jar by the door.

Let your tongue settle, wider, warmer, softer. Let your jaw drop a little toward your chest and your head bow toward the safe and comfortable space before you. Release the tension in your face and in the back of your neck. And as you take a deep breath, release your sinuses as your breath perforates your passages, channeled like steam or mist down past your palate, throat, esophagus, and into your lungs.

This relaxation is simple. It's just letting your body function naturally. You unlock the tensions in and around your chest so that your breath inflates thoroughly, evenly, and deeply beneath your sternum, below your ribs, extending broadly below the muscles of your scapula, an elastic webbing that both holds everything together and relaxes everything together, sinking into your chair, bed, sofa, armchair, hammock, carpet, moss, beach sand, floating in air, water, or space.

Now let your relaxation roll down from your neck, across your shoulders, and down your arms. And as you feel waves of relaxation notice your pulse. Maybe you feel it in your neck, chest, arms, or hands. You can feel it anywhere if you look for it, and be amazed at how absent it seems when you don't. Feel your pulse now in your hands, tolling like a metronome, and in your arms, and across your breast, pulsing above the gentler waves of breath that expand, flowing to fill, and then pause, ebb, and slack.

Scan for tension in your torso, chest, back, spine, neck, and shoulders. Tension appears as blankness, coldness, solidity, rigidity, or a furrowing, folding, inflexibility, or contraction.

It's amazing we have such poor language for tension and such limited means of describing relaxation, amazing that we have such a poor understanding of what comfort feels like, but so it is. We have no description because we have no understanding, and this is true in any language. The fault is not in our words but in our lack of awareness. This is the real object here: awareness. A perception beyond language. A body memory.

If you find some tension, and even if you don't, call back that little tractor that rumbled around your scalp and direct it to those places. Let that tractor tread back and forth over the tight spots, and if the tension is deep, then let that little tractor set its drill rig and burrow its auger into muscle, twisting and twirling the muscles as if it was stretching taffy, until that spot is loose and limp.

Focus on your hips, pelvis, sacrum, and the base of your spine. This is a place of special tensions because of the weight it carries, both as the superstructure of our posture as well as the cradle of our organs. And here, too, attach the big muscles of our buttocks and thighs, connected to the big joints of our knees, laced and cross-braced with tendons and ligaments quite a bit more vulnerable to injury than you might suspect.

Like some towering scaffold, the spine is connected to the muscles of the hips and femurs, and the big bones sit atop each other, cushioned by cartilage, meniscus, and connective tissues. These, too, need to be relaxed. The whole complex: spine, hips, pelvic floor, thighs, knees, and calves. Bring that toy tractor down to excavate the situation, to police the interior and separate the muscles down the outside of your thighs, letting your knees spread a little as warmth glows in your shins, spreading down to your ankles.

Feel the pulse in your legs. I feel it first in my thighs, but then I feel it around my thighs, and it extends down like a spear through my knees and a whisper around my calves. I don't know about you, but I carry a lot of tension in my ankles. They seem to be made of metal, as if they were artificial joints. They feel sturdy, and, indeed, I have never injured them in spite of many assaults. Perhaps yours feel more vulnerable, more like a pitchfork militia and less like an Imperial Star Cruiser. However you feel, let the pulse carry through your ankles to your feet, whether the joints pulse actively or simply resonate with the pulse around them. Move down to your feet.

Picture those foot rollers, cylindrical ridged wooden rolling pins you roll beneath your feet. Imagine them rolling under the arches of each foot, loosening the muscles in the arches and tickling the balls of your feet.

Let that little massage tractor go to work on your feet: the heels, the sides, the balls, the arches. Feel those little rolling treads forward-and-reversing over and around your feet, around each toe, and back up your Achilles tendons.

Pushing against the joints of your feet and the knuckles of your toes, feel the nerves following the tendons like upside-down tree roots, weaving around your ankles, up your shins, carrying the energies of balance, direction, and support up into the massive joints of your knees.

Feel the lighter energy coming down your legs, swaddling your feet, and launching out your toes to create roots of energy; into the ground around you, connecting your relaxation to a stability rooted in the earth itself. Real roots that keep you always connected to the ground.

Now with each breath, feel a warm sensation roll over you from head to foot, leaving a kind of tingling, more or less, in the looser sense of body, always ready to call the little massage tractor to explore the tensions you carry. Feel yourself as the liquid that you are, percolating like water through the rocks, always moving energy, nutrients, plasma, antibodies, and who knows what!

At any point you focus—calf, hip, gut, back, hand, shoulder, neck, ear, or eye—feel the natural connection, energy, and relaxation flowing through you like a river. You are a river of relaxation, waves of all heights, sounds, and frequencies, all passing through you without a sound, a turbulent concoction of attentions and emotions. All let go. All swept away. All released and relaxed. A million colored papers, all cut and mixed up like confetti, and you don't need to think about any of them. You don't need to do anything but breathe… Inhale… And exhale… letting feelings float past… Feeling clear, careless, thoughtless, and relaxed.

Let's do the count again now, and let's see if you find yourself moving into a different place as the numbers fade away. I will speak the numbers counting down from one hundred, and you will whisper beneath your breath "deeply relaxed" between each number that I count. And I'll go on for a while, until I feel the whole thing fading away.

I begin by saying, "One Hundred," and now you say, "Deeply relaxed."

Then I say, "Ninety-nine", and you say, "Deeply relaxed." And we go on…

Ninety-nine.

Ninety-eight.

Ninety-seven.

Ninety-six.

Ninety-five.

Ninety-four.

Ninety-three.

Ninety-two.

Ninety-one.

Ninety.

Let these numbers float like sensations on your skin.

Eighty-nine, Eighty-eight.

Shift your focus to the sensations beneath your skin.

Eighty-seven, Eighty-six.

A quieter and more connected world. A world of shadows and currents that we can't see clearly because we have no clear memories. We are not focusing, and we're not thinking clearly. And without focus, you become calm, because you spread out… and move into softer feelings.

Now let part of your mind come back, and let part of your mind stay

The Path to Sleep

there, like a scout, like a sentry, leaving a benchmark. Let part of you remain to remember for next time where feeling relaxed is, so that it won't take any effort to find your way back when you want to function well, without tension, with room to focus, moving toward sleep.

(Wait 30 seconds.)

And this is the end of this exercise. Return to awareness, or go further in this state, as you prefer.

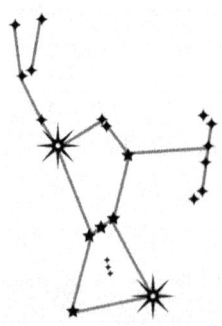

6 Mind Relaxation

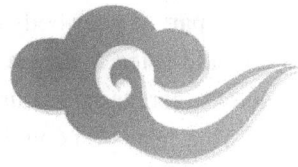

EMOTION GUIDES THE BALANCED MIND.

Building Reality

Your body is a store of memory, attitudes, postures, and relationships of past events and future expectations. Moving through your body to find relaxation is an exercise in reforming and refreshing your identity, both as the person you've grown to be and as the person you can become.

Your mind is also a store of memory, attitudes, postures, and relationships... of past events and future expectations. Moving through your mind is also an exercise... in reforming and refreshing your identity. Looking into one's mind-body is like looking into the repeating images created by two facing, parallel mirrors.

> *"Any change in the nervous system translates itself clearly through a change of attitude, posture, and muscular configuration. (The mind and the body) are not two states but two aspects of the same state."*

— Moshe Feldenkrais, engineer, physicist, physical therapist. From Moshe Feldenkrais (2010). Image, Movement, and Actor: Restoration of Potentiality. In *Embodied Wisdom: The Collected Papers of Moshe Feldenkrais*. Berkeley, CA: North Atlantic Book.

Our preconception of difference between mind and body comes from our experience with injury, recovery, and in our maintenance of balance. Because a brain injury affects our thinking and a foot injury affects our walking, we assert thinking is in the brain and walking is in the foot. But is it really? Many brain injuries affect your walking and foot injuries affect your thinking. There are repeated stories of heart transplant recipients whose new lives follow the old trajectory of their heart's donor.

Imagine how you might move differently and feel differently about your body if you really understood each part of your body as part of your identity. How much more carefully you would listen to the pressures in your chest, the grumblings of your stomach, and the soreness in your feet if you knew that those tissues authored a voice in your head you could not live without?

People are what they think and become the stories they believe, but they don't recognize this because it is too fluid. They prefer an external reality, as if reality is cast in a mold. This mold defines a boundary of what is inside and outside of us. Believing in this creates a "me" and a "them," a good and a bad, a victim and a perpetrator, the guilty and the innocent, right and wrong. These are the beliefs we accept as the basis for probity, virtue, society, and sanity.

Most people most of the time, and some people all of the time, fail to recognize this as a creation, something we call consensual reality, and this is why people can't relax. Because if they did, the world might fall apart. Is it why you can't relax?

> *"We are in many ways driven about by external causes, and that like waves of the sea driven by contrary winds we toss to and fro unwitting of the issue and of our fate."*
>
> — Benedict de Spinoza (1632 – 1677). From *The Ethics*, Translated by R. H. M. Elwes.

Insomnia

Insomnia is a cognitive dysfunction related to a neurochemical imbalance, they are two aspects of the same thing. Many of my insomniac clients take over-the-counter or prescription medication to promote sleep. This has not cured them, but it often promotes some relaxation.

These people's insomnia will be cured when they learn to deeply relax, which says nothing about how to achieve it. Most chronic insomniacs cannot relax, and some refuse to try because relaxation is not part of their character.

Because I work with people's minds, I address insomnia cognitively, but insomnia also has a somatic component. Tension released from the mind only to be stored in the body is tension retained. Sweeping tension under your structural carpet will not cure insomnia. However, it's likely that carrying tension in your body has become such a habit that you no longer know it's there. You will need to explore it in order to uncover and release it.

I can talk many of my tense, insomniac clients to sleep using guided visualizations. They will follow my words, but they cannot use their own. This is evidence that while we communicate verbally and can share the same thoughts, our minds do not run on the same rails. Our minds inhabit different emotional landscapes, and those landscapes are poorly described by words.

Let's say your emotional landscape is how you feel about what you think, and this landscape prevents your moving into sleep. You would like to divest yourself of these aggravating emotions, but you cannot. And this is because the purpose of emotions is to orient you, to direct your focus. You cannot easily ignore what you are directed toward.

"What if the underlying problem is NOT that you can't fall asleep... what if there were another, greater part of you that is trying to help you symbolically wake up?"

—Dr. Cara Barker, Jungian Analyst

Sleep problems are life problems. You cannot discard them. You must deal with them. The issues that arise when you try to relax are wounds that need your attention. Consider words to be ineffective—after all, you've been using words your whole life and your problems remain.

Imagine that you are hunting for solutions. You must track them down. Your emotions are these tracks and you must follow them. If you're not good at putting emotions into words, or, more likely, you don't want to, then you've got to track your quarry by following clues that only you can discern. To do this, you must look at your emotions. You must "wake up" to your feelings. Your insomnia is not the problem. Your insomnia is your being on the trail to your solution. What you need to do is hunt, not sleep. The problem is that you're not following the trail.

"She was cured (of her insomnia) by the grace of God... How was I to tell him that I had sung her a lullaby with my mother's voice? Enchantment like that is the oldest form of medicine..."

— Carl Jung, 1959. From Duplain, G. (1987). The Frontiers of Knowledge. In William McGuire & R. F. C. Hull (Eds.), *C. G. Jung Speaking: Interviews and Encounters* (pp. 410-423). Princeton, NJ: Princeton University Press.

Identity

The mind and body are not so separate. Certain organs do certain things, and it only makes sense that tissues carry memory, reaction, and inclination. Think of injury, scarring, growth, and exercise. Scars of a major injury would, and perhaps have, had major effects on your view of self, your presentation of yourself, and what you think. Think of childbirth, think of endurance.

Does the body just provide a reminder through sensation, or is it a repository of memory? The sensible answer is both. Each affects the other. Each exists within the other. The picture of the body as the vehicle and the mind as the driver may work for navigating the landscape, but it does not work for navigating ourselves. The body thinks. The body remembers. And when the body speaks, we interpret it as coming from the mind.

Years ago my friend and I beached our windsurfing boards on an unfamiliar shore of a large Texas lake. We found ourselves invited to beer and burgers by a posse of relaxed Texas bubbas, and their well-manicured wives and kids. The sky was blue, the water warm, and our gracious hosts were attired for the hot afternoon in cowboy boots, wide-brimmed hats, and not so much as a stitch of clothing between them.

That friendly encounter remains my paradigm of Texas thinking: "We do it our way, and you can like it… or you can leave!" We had a lovely time, noting nothing out of the ordinary, before sailing off into the sunset. It's all in the thinking, and how you accept it. There is no "normal" outside of how others define it and you react to it.

Could you let go of yourself so much that your friends wouldn't recognize you? Could you let yourself go so far that you wouldn't know who you were anymore? Would you feel safe? Safe knowing that you can always reassemble yourself later, after you've taken your skin off and washed the sand out.

"Absence" is a short exercise aimed at letting go, and let's watch ourselves doing this, and watch how you watch yourself, and how you stop yourself from slipping over the edge to... to what?

Let me remind myself of where we're going. We're building visions of who we might be, have once been, or are moving to become that will allow us to relax. And relax is our word meaning "all things possible with no tension on our part," as in "recreate," "restore," and "revitalize."

I want to build a world of imagination that has a rich texture and no baggage, something that can generate a different awareness, one to which you can return. Something both familiar and unfamiliar, that carries no triggers, or reminders of things you want to leave behind.

The next exercise, called "Ascent," is a story of a place you've never been, unlike any place you *have* been, partly recalled and partly invented as a doorway to open your imagination.

Perhaps you've had experiences that resonate with this story, so you can be there, too. And that's what I want, for you to create a memory with *your* imagination that is at the same time so present and so distant that you can be in both places at once.

To remind you of why we're at this point: we aim to relax the mind as a way to create relaxation in the body. Relaxing the mind lies in the realm of ideas. I present "Absence" to explore the idea that you can lose yourself in pictures of disintegration into rain, and wind, air, and energy. Replace your idea of yourself with ideas of emptiness. These are ideas that take up mental space as opposed to mental emptiness, which your waking mind finds unnatural and refills with the usual stuff.

"Ascent" presents mental pictures evocative of things familiar but disconnected or disconnectable from the normal cues and triggers that attach your armored self to its tourniquets of tension and tattoos of concern. Join me in an experience that wears away and then reconnects your mind with a perfection so thin it has to be imagined.

These are substitutions. The first, relaxing in the sun. The second, a bedtime story. I'm not asking you to remember them but to feel where they take you. If you relax, remember *that* feeling because, while I told the story, you made the change. If you know how to make the change, you don't need the story.

Listen to these stories as much as you want with the goal of not needing them. Develop new balance and flexibility so you can reach relaxation in an instant.

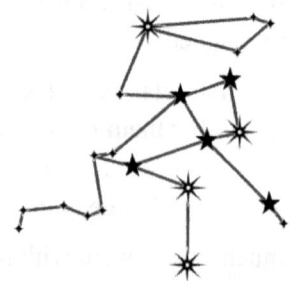

Hypnotic Session 11

Absence

Audio file at: https://www.mindstrengthbalance.com/path-to-sleep-audio/

Lie back, close your eyes, and find a relaxed pose, arms at your sides or folded over you. Feeling comfortable, place your attention between your eyes, somewhere at your forehead. Tell yourself your eyelids are heavy, like velvet theater curtains with chain links woven into the hem, locking them down, lightless and relaxed, inert and insensate. Stand back beyond the empty auditorium of your eyelids, feeling entirely uninterested in looking.

Move above yourself, beyond and outside yourself. See yourself shrouded in a mist, silver, gold, or white. This mist tumbles and churns, folding in over your head, and twisting 'round your limbs like a vortex, slowly rotating around your body, emanating from your head, twisting, enveloping, encircling each arm and each leg separately, and folding back into itself below you to continue its electric cycle, passing through you.

Listen to the world around you, and imagine that you can hear the ticking of a clock. If it is daytime imagine, you can hear the singing of a bird. If it is nighttime, imagine the hooting of an owl. Imagine the sound of a train double-clicking somewhere far away, fading into the distance. Imagine the sound of a windy rain with the drops incessantly tapping on the window.

Feel the weight of your shoulders and let your shoulders… drop. Let your arms feel light, and then lighter, and then lifting up, as if they're floating up at your sides, weightless. Feel the weight of your lower back pressing down on your pelvis and hips. Imagine this weight released, so that back and pelvis are no longer pressing down. You still feel the sensation of weight, but your legs, and thighs, and feet feel lighter. Push them, stretch them, and wiggle your toes so that your feet relax, light and energized.

You are no longer anchored to the floor but are elevated, as if parts of you are attached to balloons taking the force of gravity away. Let your body awareness float a few feet up above where your body sits or lies. Even as you stretch or move your body, feeling the chair or bed around you, you can still feel the sense of floating, supported by nothing but the air around you.

Take a deep breath, hold it for an instant, and as you exhale imagine your chest punched full of holes and the air you exhale leaks out from all sides. And as you inhale, the air pours in through all the holes in your chest... and back out again as you exhale.

Your body is floating in the middle of the room, supported by a hundred balloons. Your chest is full of holes, and your breath inflates and deflates through the Swiss cheese of your skin. Your awareness slips out of your body as the air slips out of your lungs, and with each beat of your heart, dissolve into the air like sugar stirred into hot water, the crystals becoming fewer and fewer, and the steam exiting the surface to be torn to tatters, wisps whisked into a moist air, as your spirit and awareness diffuse through the room around you.

Hear the moan of a distant truck engine, or maybe it's an airplane or the blood pulsing in your ears, and let your awareness ooze through the walls of the house or building you're in, until you find yourself swirling around it like flakes in a snow globe, anchored to the house or building at the center of your vortex. Once around... Twice around... Now let that vortex go, and disassemble yourself out even further, out beyond the house into the trees, beyond the building, into the air swirling among other blocks, into the updrafts where the hawks, crows, and seagulls fly.

A crow comes flying past, rowing its wings, scanning with its jet black eye. It sees you for an instant, gives a penetrating glare before shooting past in its fast pace on strong currents. And you feel yourself scattered by the wind, blown to shreds to tumble, looking up into the sky and down into the labyrinth of tracks and treetops.

And you become the sky with nothing but the sensation of air around you, with no sensation of anything inside you, simply taking up space without dimension—a flag torn free of its banner like a jet of smoke or a streamer shot from a cannon, rippling sensations sweeping over your body as you feather almost weightless down... down through the sky... down toward the Earth.

And as you fall, weightless, backwards, easy, you become a raindrop. First, small as a drizzle, and then growing larger, catching other small, clear specs of water growing to a drop, undulating in the air, falling like a little package, smooth and silvery, reflecting all the world in your circular mirror, down toward the place you sit or lie.

Passing through the air, a glint of light on a buffet of breeze that makes the trees sway, strike the corner of the window, leaving a long track, writing all your sky memories in the meandering water down the window pane. Back to your place, floating in this room, back into your body, held together with elastic and memories.

Reform your spine and arms and legs of a stick figure, build your flesh and bones, coming back into sight like the restoration of the invisible man: first bones, then veins and nerves, capillaries and tissues, muscles, joints, skin wrapping around your body, encircling your limbs and digits, unrolling across your face and around your scalp.

Now recall you're lying or sitting here but not feeling exactly the same, now slightly... disjointed. The nuts and bolts are loosened. Not that anything is rattling or rolling, but no longer clamped, cramped, locked, or bound—in a boneless way, as if your bones had all turned to cartilage. Like an octopus, you're all sense and nonsense, able to reform at whim, to squeeze through the smallest hole, to fill and to fit any container.

In particular, the container of sleep holds you like ingredients in measuring cups, ready to be mixed, battered, and stirred until all the lumps are out, poured and percolated into a soft cake, steaming and settling with deflation... inflation... and deflation, back toward the forms of sleep. Anytime your body tells you to fall in, fall out, and return to a hundred fingers of sleep. Re-leavened in body, and re-dissolved of mind.

Sleep now. Sleep now, off like a cardboard box on a conveyor belt of rollers. Boxes upon boxes. Focus folded upon focus, wrapped up in series and parallel, in a moment enduring, extent and instant. Sifted and flowing

The Path to Sleep

like a powder, like smoke, like an open window letting your mind out to wander and consider… anything.

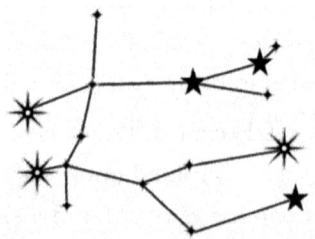

Hypnotic Session 12

Ascent

Audio file at: https://www.mindstrengthbalance.com/path-to-sleep-audio/

Mountains are symbols of achievement and a metaphor for the unattainable, and we're aiming to achieve the unattainable, so let's go climb a mountain. Let's climb a big one. Let's go deep into the wilderness and climb a peak that's rarely seen. There aren't any trails, and there are hardly any roads, so we'll have to make our own way.

There are places in the Rocky Mountains where people rarely go. The valleys are empty, and the country is wild. Shingled rivers saw the occasional trapper or prospector, but those days are gone. Today, logging and oil companies fly past, looking for stands, rifts, and faults. In the valleys where they find them, they'll sweep through like marauders, but the alpine country is ignored. Above the valley, we'll see nothing of them or of anyone. There are still places humans have never been, mountains that haven't changed in a million years.

I've got a map with contours drawn by satellites, tripoded by splintered rivers set in shadings of deep green. Green gives way to gray where the trees begin to grumble, then white where perennial snows shelter between the buttresses, and black where nothing else holds on. Let's go and see what's up there: mountain lions, Bigfoot, or specters of ourselves.

We travel by mind, so settle in for the journey on an astral trip to a place that does exist and which you will someday encounter, at least in spirit. Find a comfortable chair or bed and strap in like an astronaut for launch. Take a breath. Inhale and exhale. Relax. When your vision clears and your heartbeat settles, we'll be ready. Take that extra effort to clear all systems, to relax all tension. Close your eyes with all systems go, and we'll start the countdown:

Ten, nine, eight. Let yourself feel the shudder of the rockets of your imagination.

The Path to Sleep

Seven, six, five. Clear a tunnel opening up in front of you.

Four, three, two. There's a tapping as the doors of your perception are unlatched.

And one. And with a gentle acceleration that is both soft and comfortable, imagine that someone has taken off the parking brake and the wagon of your mind starts to roll. Let it roll, sway, and float into that tunnel of sensation, of sparkles and shooting stars behind your eyelids as we soar on a trajectory, like a baseball struck by a giant, through the air to arc above the present world, launched into the wild blue yonder.

Let clouds streak past with a whooshing noise inside your ears, and, like Jack who's climbed the beanstalk, imagine a new landscape passing below you, as unreal as looking out the porthole of an airplane, but now there is no airplane, only you in your mind's eye, flying like a spaceship from another civilization above a wooded landscape, lush with haze and shadows, giddy with distance far below. Take a breath. Inhale… Exhale. And relax into the descent.

The rockets have jettisoned, the heat dissipates, and our parachutes have deployed. Let things seem quiet, and imagine hearing only a rush as our elevation deflates with the hiss of air between our ears, and the world settles vertically. Everything is still now and brilliant in the shocking silver sunlight, as we move toward Earth, downward, into the gullet of the horizon, being swallowed back to home as the encircling Earth receives us. More real than just imagination, felt ancestrally in your bones. Back to ground, back to Earth, back to the center of the Earth.

And then, as if from nowhere, forested land appears below us, and then, with such short notice, trees and treetops—with the dizzying wash of space between them. And then we're between them, and then they're beside us, rising up, and before we can feel them, we can hear them. In a raspy, tearing, snapping of branches, in a confetti of snapped twigs and torn leaves, we're dumped without ceremony in a clearing between two pines, on a hillock in the creek valley of some river we can't see.

With the insight of imagination, we know we're heading up and into the woods, as the benefit of gravity reminds us with untiring indication. You've got a pack, and you've got boots, clothes slightly rumpled and a little overweight, perhaps, but none the worse for wear. Cutting free from the shrouds, roll up the 'chute that held us, and bury it snugly beneath the rocks, apologizing that we can't pack it out, and head off toward the creek.

What our navigation lacks in details it makes up for in enthusiasm and the wonder of the brilliant day. To be in a place of total quiet and seclusion, as you rarely find in life. It may be a bit too sunny, but it holds deep shadows, waiting for our introduction.

Off we go on a bushwhacking adventure. You remember adventure? It's what you do when you're feeling bored with life. It's as simple as taking a new turn, stepping into an unknown building, or greeting a stranger. Recall that feeling now, except all turns are new, everything is unknown, and there is nothing you have seen before. The rocks are somewhat unusual and even the trees look a bit strange. Following the sloping banks, we push into the snagging bush, looking for the creek whose flowing waters could lead us—even in total blindness—into the high country.

The land is big, and the vistas would be grand if we could see farther than mice amid towering fir trees. Imagine gliding between mountains, but all we can do is navigate between tree trunks. Do you turn into this brush-clogged tumble or that exuberant wall of bramble? Both riots of rooted vegetation refuse our passage with indignance, pointing instead to the creek's prattling waterway. There, at least, the roots are shallow and the gravel always shifting. The creek's wet passage would be welcome except for a million young branches erupting from the banks to grab the sunlight sparkling off silver-black water.

Trackless land is rough with silt and vegetation, leaf-covered holes between boulders the millennia have washed down from the forested hillside. You can see straight forward but cannot travel straight by any means. The exhausting heaving, clamoring, and circumambulation of the sloping hillside points over its shoulder for the simple creek bed which, though clogged with branches and slipping stones, offers an endless chain of watery planes linked by flower-crusted clumps of weeds.

It's a lot of work, but, given enough time and effort, we can look back on accomplishing a hundred feet of passage, and with another hour, another few hundred feet, and eventually, as the day wears on, the valley envelops us between steepening walls, which, although we don't feel much further, definitely make us feel much deeper into a landscape of splintered wood and rock-chiseled teeth.

Let's call it a day, and, if we're lucky, we'll find a place to lie down. It feels like resting on a battlefield with obstacles all around us. We find a large and senior tree, old enough to have shaped the land and hushed the undergrowth beneath its skirts. Standing up puts branches in our face, but lying down offers a carpet of twigs and old needles. Lay out a pad and sleeping bag, and crawl in with your jacket as a pillow.

Ironic that you've come for the air sweeping across towering walls, and now you find yourself curled up amidst the roots of life in a moist tree cavern. And there, quite exhausted, a few pointed sticks are no obstacles to an entirely peaceful, boundless sleep.

Waking under the canopy of a deep valley—it would be dimly lit, even at high noon—sleeping with the sunset assures waking before sunrise. Filtered morning light drizzles from a pinkening sky, and your body is quite sore, all the more-so for the sharp sticks that you paid no heed, but left their impression. You aren't used to sleeping in any dimple you can find, so it feels good to return to the goal-oriented world of novelty and progress.

Yet this day is pretty much the same as the last, perhaps with walls a bit steeper and water a bit faster, less soil and more rock cut into sluices rather than built as walls. The endless novelty becomes repetitive: wet socks and slippings, squishing boots the norm. Only the special puzzles you remember: as when the creek opened to an uncrossably deep pool, or high walls maked unwalkable water-rushes you had to climb around. Choose between wading cold, fast waters, or jungle-gymming algae-slicked, sharp and broken branch-studded tree trunks. Leveling-up through one challenge after another, challenges small but serious, stumbling unheroically against moss, mud, and water pressure.

So passes another day, with slower progress past more obstacles, with more scratches and greater exertion so that, come the late afternoon, you're even more tired than the day before. And you're wetter with even less to show for it, and there are fewer flat places. It's one of those far too long and exciting days, leaving you to ask if you're having fun yet. The setting sun rings the closing bell.

You do not regret in the least throwing in the towel, happy for any chance to sit down. You could sleep anywhere, and you do, grateful for another dozen hours that will pass with the blink of your exhausted eyes. Remember those days now, whether they were physically or emotionally exhausting. Days when you could discard your clock schedule for nature's downtime sun-cycle.

Close your imaginary eyes, and take a break from everything, glad to be safe and to forget, and there is no one to remind you as the entire force of nature bags you off to sleep. Ahh, for the simple pleasure of taking your shoes off… and sleep until dawn.

Nature is episodic. Things go on until they stop, and when they stop, they stop suddenly. River banks, treetops, forests that stop at the tree line, and this creek-choked odyssey that ends quite suddenly when the trees defer to a climate that gets too cold. So, too, the grasses and weeds abandon soil that's just a bit too dry and thin, and the landscape changes suddenly from thick forest to boulder slopes. The burbling brook descends out of earshot into groundwater tunnels carved through shale and boulder fields, and all you're left to hear are the whistling sounds of wind playing Aeolian pipes on a drying, bare, and climbing landscape.

All you have is a selfie of yourself having emerged from that chaos creek of sundews and salamanders—insignificant but for its endlessness—looking like the survivor of some beer-house brawl, punch-drunk and swollen-faced, having stepped on and been hit by one too many garden rakes.

Have you ever recalled good memories from uncomfortable times? It seems possible there are two sets of memories, one set pleasant and the other not, as if they happened at different times or to separate people. Maybe you had a wonderful trip but got sick or had a great visit to an injured relative. A single event with two points of view, and you can choose to remember one and forget the other. Sometimes the prize comes at the end of a sharp stick. We're good at seeing opposites, so consider what miseries are still attached to the things you're really grateful for.

Finally, on this third day, we can see the river, embedded in its green-way, snaking down below us as we transition to the alpine. Ahead, now foreshortened by our mountain's enormous shoulders, are fields of crocodile-, pink-, and seaweed-colored lichens stretching to a water-colored smear into even more stark mountains beyond.

Our vegetable thrashing relents, thankfully, into boulder scrambling, which, because they're large and old, don't shift much beneath our weight. It's a metamorphosis, as if we've emerged from grubbing through the brush to dance on spindly legs up rising fields of ancient rocks. We've reached treeline, a point where the seeds, soils, and temperature don't satisfy the forest. It stops quite suddenly, the forest's upper edge pushed back like a cuticle by slides of summer rock and winter snow. And the light changes, and the air changes, and your thoughts change to find a new gait, movement, and stream of mind.

You know, the worst thing about exertion is when you can't find your pace, but here you can. Your breath and pulse balance the strain and effort, and you maintain a steady pace. The shifting footing demands attention, but, as if with blindsight, you can see it without thinking, and there is a corner of your mind that's free to think, but, in spite of this, there is not much to think about.

You try to think about your problems, anxious situations, and uncertainties of the future, things you carry like rocks in your gizzard. You try, but it's like pouring out ball bearings, and they just won't stay put. And no sooner than you try to worry, they're washed away into a huge horizon and the miles of space all around you, falling away by gravity without an echo.

Above you are the tops of ancient valleys, loose ridges piled with stones left by long-gone glaciers, melted under this same warm sun and sky. The boulder slope is like a broken escalator, half a mile long. The steps are too high, and many are missing entirely.

Each step offers a puzzle-choice, placing your feet on twisted treads, which your turning mind resolves with the pace of each footstep. Inhale, step… Step… Exhale, step… Step… You would lose interest except for the risk of breaking your pace or twisting your ankle. Progress is steady, slow, and cadenced with your breath. The endless slope is hypnotic: Inhale, step… Step… Exhale, step… Step… And whenever you look up, you find yourself a little higher. Black, chiseled peaks slowly emerge in profile against the crowns of snow-white slopes, a hall of mountain kings.

Long slopes go on forever, foreshortened distances that are hard to judge. Every bump hides what's beyond and looks like the top… until you get past it and find the slope keeps going on the other side, but you feel the change as it gets easier in your legs. The sky seems to be getting larger when you look at it—which isn't often, as your feet take all your attention—but you're breathing easier and have more freedom to think. You're almost able to change your pace but that would mess up your cadence, so you just feel lighter. Time goes a little faster, and other ideas pass through your mind—ideas related and unrelated, nose to the grindstone, dreams of future comfort.

Running through a field… Inhale… Step… Step… Exhale… Step… Step.

Swinging in a hammock… Inhale… Step… Step… Exhale… Step… Step.

Walking on a driftwood beach… Inhale… Step… Step… Exhale… Step… Step.

Daydream images flaking past like autumn leaves, floating in your mind, settling in your memory. What do you believe in?

The Path to Sleep

High above peaks we barely remember, with the creek hidden in velvet green snaking below our feet, we scramble into a gentle swale, stumbling onto flat ground, feeling like falling forward with nothing to resist us.

We're on a high shoulder, a sort of viewing platform, leading down to a pass with a background of secondary peaks too low to pierce the horizon, the hazy chasms darkening in the late afternoon. Evening rises up from the valleys like a fog, as if intending to approach us, and our eyes are tired of looking, and it's all too far away to matter.

Here is a shallow pond, spring-fed with a sandy beach, ruffed by a garden of Paintbrush, Fireweed, and white Asters. We roll the small boulders, filling their holes with dust and sand to make a perfect campsite, feeling silly it's so easy since there are no trees or roots to hold the soil. Dropping off to valleys on three sides below. A weary, sighing sky. A reddening western sun.

Drop your pack to feel light-footed, and walk barefoot as if it's no big deal. At the world's top, a few clouds slumber past, and with nothing to do, you soak your feet, sitting in the sand amidst the flowers. If you could be satisfied with perfection, you'd go no further, but perfection is never enough. Is a feeling enough if you can't own it, hold it, or put in the bank? Let an image of this spot be etched into your mind, a place so perfect you can't appreciate it.

It seems that no one's been here before, as there is no trace or path, just rocks and flowers, light, air, and space. Lots of space, probably as much space as you'll ever find, miles in all directions, including down. And the light is special because, with so much sky, everything is lit up all day, a solarium from dawn to twilight, while the dark valleys, eroding ever deeper, wetter, and more fertile, soak up light as they soak up water, giving the feeling that to look down is to look inside yourself.

Must it take three days and a vertical mile to get here, at this perfect spot at the end of the world? A warm sun, a few bees, a shallow pond. A perfect meadow surrounded by perfect air and perfect light. To sit comfortably among flowers in the biggest IMAX auditorium on Earth, to watch the solar hour hand's singular melodrama sweep across the sky.

It's a virtual reality, a state of mind I call you into. A state of rising above it all, yet we can never remain here for long. And that's just what perfect relaxation is: to have moved above all struggle and to be in a place where you just can't seem to stay for long.

And here you are, holding your newborn mind in the palms of your hands, thinking, "So what do I do now?" And you don't really know, and it doesn't really matter because the event is over. You've reborn yourself, and now it's just another struggle to the next level of disembodiment, to the next rebirth, to more light and more air.

And here ends "the approach," and from here you can begin the climb to summit these various peaks. And it has happened before, as it happened here, that what you'll remember most is just getting here, birthing the reality that took so much effort to conceive, which, from this point, moves on without much intention. From here, you just paint by numbers to one summit or another, following the lines of gullies and ridges until there is no more "up" to go. A simple process toward simple goals.

The whole affair is somewhat akin to a fish jumping out of its bowl. It's pathetic, really, this fishbowl analogy. It's not the leap that's liberating so much as realizing the bowl is an illusion in what is really a boundless sea. Fish are fish, and so are you, and it's not about getting higher but getting bigger.

Get above your fishbowl and look around. You can do that now. There is so much air and light. Every lungful of this hologram is an ocean you've never explored if you can only sense its presence, as you can only do by relaxing to receive what you have nowhere to put, and you can't stay there for long because fish breathe water, and you must have your air, and air will take you back down into the forest.

For that moment, as long as you can give yourself, you can feel what you are now and might or can be, a membrane between states of consciousness, and when you're ready, you'll push again until, at some point, your struggles to relax will birth another form in your adamant ascent from fishhood to

The Path to Sleep

whatever we are to become.

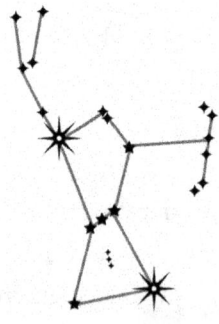

7 Comfort

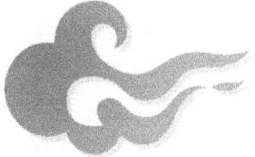

LEARNING TO BE COMFORTABLE IS A SKILL.

Pain

Pain is an altered state, one you can learn to intercept and redirect. With self-control you can reduce pain by half and, with practice, you may eliminate it entirely. Normal people have done amazing things when necessary, with focus and with help.

I don't know why some people are more adept than others. In my experience, altering your state is more a matter of overcoming the fear of letting go than creating distance. You are not naturally closely bound to your senses; you bind yourself to your senses. If you can relax those bonds, you naturally separate from your body and its senses.

Let's talk a little about what pain is, because it's not as straightforward as you might think. First, there is anxiety. It's not so clear what this has to do with pain, though by itself it is uncomfortable.

Anxiety is an expectation and an amplifier. Anxiety is a pain trigger, and it can set pain off, even when there is nothing painful. As a child, my father's friends would blindfold and burn each other… with ice cubes. If you are sure you're about to be burned by something, then just about anything harsh that touches you will burn, even an ice cube.

The point is, pain is what your brain manufacturers, and while it's usually triggered by a trauma or injury, it can be triggered by your imagination, and it can hurt just as much. There are cases where a plain, dull, cool stick raised a burn-like welt through nothing more, apparently, than expectation.

I'm not saying your pain is imaginary. I'm saying that pain is an image, and you must have an image before you'll feel anything. You cannot control a trauma or injury, but you can control your images of them. This is especially important when you are magnifying this image and making the pain bigger. There is no one-to-one; there is no such thing as a non-amplified pain. This process of making an image is something we all do in our own ways. It may be out of your control now, but it is within your control eventually. Don't feel guilty about it. You have no choice but to perceive pain, but you do have a choice in how you perceive it.

Anxiety is the lock, and your intention is the key. Stand back and consider what your pain means to you. All its history. All its worry and fear. The monster that jumps out startles you, and you fear it before you see it.

There is an aspect of your pain that's fear based. Your anticipation creates its own pain that hurts when triggered by fear. Yes, it's in your head, but yes, it's also real pain. And yes, once this fear is triggered, you are undefended, arms open, inviting the sensation that follows, and that pain is the pain you fear.

This is important. Do not prejudge pain. Do not be afraid of a sensation. Do not make things worse. If you flinch or tremble, stare, sweat, or stutter, then you're anxious. Your discomfort at watching your blood being drawn is an example: it doesn't really hurt, but watching it does. Be it an injection or a torn-off band-aid, the anticipation is often more painful than the real sensation. That's the point: sensations are not entirely "real." They are partially imagined.

Separation

This is a course on sleep, and sleep is a natural separation. If you are having trouble with sleep, perhaps you need help separating from your senses. Do not think that you cannot do it. You can, and much of what we've explored regarding sleep will help: rhythms, intention, self-connection, broader horizons, and subtle perception.

Reframing is a place to start. You are not disconnecting from discomfort; you are connecting to comfort. But you must find it first. You must look away from that which engulfs, demands, and obsesses you. Discomfort is a form of obsession. Anything that is not an option is a kind of obsession, even if you're helpless before it. Look for the ties that bind you. You will find a long legacy hidden in places you have not looked.

Before reframing, accept responsibility. Accept responsibility for disease, for comfort, for sleep, for your life. That does not mean that you like it or that you can change it. It means that you admit you created it, if not consciously, then through the ninety-nine percent of the you that is unconscious. Taking responsibility is admitting that you will endeavor to see into that invisible ninety-nine percent.

Responsibility is a state of determination—and maybe hope—but more likely faith, faith in yourself. This is what most of us lack: faith in ourselves. We have been taught to abandon ourselves. It's what our asset-based culture demands. We are stripped, showered, reclothed, and sent to work. Regaining faith is abandoning the culture of need. You cease following the light and become the light. It has always been this way. That is the path to all your healing.

There is nothing wrong with feeling, being, or having been a victim, but if you persist then you must take responsibility for it. If not, then reject that role. The victim, like the student, is a learner, and you graduate when school offers no more value.

The student role is weak, condescended below the rank of practitioner. The perpetual student is not a perpetual learner, but they may be a perpetual victim. In healing, as in all exploration, be your own teacher, and learn from the richness of your own mistakes. Entering uncharted waters, you become an expert.

You may think you have nothing to teach. You may think no one is interested. That is the student-victim talking. In their lifetimes— you may be surprised to know—Dante, Da Vinci, Newton, and Einstein found few were interested in what they really thought. They worked alone and, to a large degree, lived alone. That's why they got so far.

If you hope to find insight then you must take a solitary path and accept some of the same fate of being isolated. The irony is that as explorers, they would not have traded their solitude for anything. Once you meet yourself as loving guide, you will not forsake your solitude, either.

Only you can teach you. Don't expect a grade, pill, certificate, silver bullet, or gold star. Expect to fail and fail gleefully, because with each failure, you raise yourself a notch. And don't worry about failing the same way twice. There is no such thing.

> *"As I get older, I realize being wrong isn't a bad thing like they teach you in school. It is an opportunity to learn something."*
>
> — R.P. Feynman, physicist (1918-1988)

Remain aware, stretch to your limit, and, as they say in athletics, "feel the burn." That's what your discomfort is, so rest at ease. You are at your edge. Stay there, be patient, do the work, and you will change.

Separating from sensation is not hard, but it is disconcerting. Sort of like levitating yourself, it can make you quite anxious to look down on the nail points of sensations. Fear is the main obstacle to believing that you can fly above it, a flight that is real as long as you can imagine it. It takes practice. Practice not so much to do it as to believe that you can and that you can hold it. After all, if you were just learning to levitate, would you stray above any terrain harder than a hay stack? Not likely.

Joints

Comfort is a general thing, built on being free of pain and anxiety. But discomfort, as comes from pain, is specific, and addressing it may require being specific. The exercise "Disconnection" aims to be general and nonspecific enough to encompass different people's issues, but if you have a specific issue, I would like to address it. I would like to go the extra mile to reach you and not require you to use a one-size-fits-all prescription.

Unfortunately, I can't. I can't lead you to marshal resources for every ache and worry. There are too many, and every pang means something special and often quite different to each person. Just consider the anxieties of a group of people subject to the same distress. Each person will likely have a different reaction and presentation. While it's true passengers on a rough sea may all get seasick, their underlying associations will differ, and the work we're doing here acts essentially at these underlying levels.

This is not a book on pain relief, only a chapter, so I must pick something general enough to be widely shared and specific enough to be a useful example, so I pick joints. We've all got them, and by the nature of aging, use, exercise, infection, and injury we all experience joint problems sooner or later and more or less.

Joint pain is familiar, though not uniform. There are muscle, bone, skin, cartilage, tendon, and ligament issues. Swelling, circulation, and degradation lead to immobility, scarring, and deformation. But still, the pain of joint discomfort is a hot, graveled, dull, or shooting pain. So let's address this kind of pain specifically. We won't care where it is, be it a worn-out knee or chronic arthritis. I want to present a short visualization to relieve joint pain of all sorts.

Separating Ideas

Separating is a form of dissociating, separating from parts of yourself. This is useful for something like pain. You can take this skill another step and separate from your thinking mind, your agitation, that rigid sense of self and worry that prevents exfolding into dreamtime. Separate by shaking loose, by turning from front to back, inside to outside, small to wide, back to front, forward to backward, back and forth, weakening your normal self's hold on reality a little more each time.

The exercise "Painless Joints" sounds much different from the first, but it is the next step—taking dissociation into the idea realm and from sensation to ideation. That is the exercise: a story that dissolves, removes, or discards things. Replace some ideas with other ideas, and let feelings follow. Become big enough to leave behind the linear, and take another form.

Comfort is a noun and a state of mind, not an adjective that describes it. It all happens in our mind, shaped and enabled by our state. We've talked about getting your mind out from under physical pain, and this is hard to talk about in a way that makes sense. It's easier done than said.

If you have issues of discomfort, sensations, sounds, or thoughts that disturb you, visualize your gradual prominence and command over them. Practice replacing, reframing, redefining, and re-experiencing them. Only you can do it, and you can do it more easily than you think.

You don't need to succeed completely at first. Just do what you can, and learn what you can do. Then do more, and accept and admire the gaining of your power over issues and events that you have so externalized, events that you've been told to externalize, as if you could never have control. You can redefine, and you can internalize, and from there you have as much control as you're willing to learn.

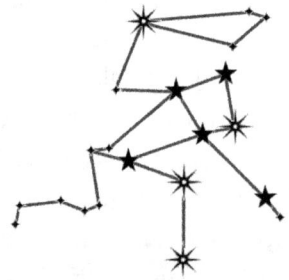

Hypnotic Session 13

Disconnection

Audio file at: https://www.mindstrengthbalance.com/path-to-sleep-audio/

If you have pain, it's time to release it. And if you don't have pain, then release it anyway, because pain is just overbearing presence, and I want to teach you to leave all presence, of any bearing, behind you.

Pain stops sleep like getting your coat tail caught in a revolving door. It doesn't need to be painful, and it's not really the pain but the connection it creates. Of course, pain is a message, but we normally "get it" well enough, and getting sleep is really what we need.

In fact, we're left to wonder, if sleep is healing, why we don't we get more of it? Why won't whoever is leaning on that klaxon let off so that we can get more of it? Isn't that what pain wants? Healing? Apparently not. Pain is self-centered. It's all about the pinching, swelling, pressing. And because pain isn't smart enough to know what's good for it and to recognize you're doing your best, we must learn to shut its mouth for it. Heartless it may be, as the masses are still suffering, but for the healing we need the sleep more than just to bear the pain.

And I assume you've done your best, and even so, perhaps you ought to have a private talk with pain. Inquire if pain has anything more to say beyond the senses. Before you turn if off, before you pull the plug and cut the wires, be aware that you're not cutting the power. The trigger is still there, triggering, and the cause still causing. Silencing pain is not pulling the fuse as the short circuit will remain. It's just turning down the volume and leaving the room.

Connection

You have to connect before you can disconnect. We're performing a kind of surgery here, a psychic surgery, and we need to know what it is we are removing. But don't be frightened, because what you will see is what you can heal, all within the range of your ability. It must be of course. Why would we want to imagine anything more? Well, actually, there are reasons for that as well, as that is the path of healing, but the path of relief is much simpler. Relief is simply taking the thorn out and calming everyone down. Healing is something else, and let this alone be a relief to you and make your task easier.

Many listening to me will not have pain, but do not feel left out. You can make it just to unmake it, and, if the truth be told, we all have pain all the time. We just call it normal, and we ignore it. This is true. Next time you have an ache or pain, something as simple as shifting in your seat, don't do it. Focus on the discomfort, and let it remain. Water it, and, like flowers, it will grow. Just as you can tune down pain, so you can increase it. And you can increase it anywhere, anytime. A masochist's dream! So join us. You may need this skill someday. I'm certain you will.

Focus on a pain, and if it isn't exactly a pain, then focus on a sensation. Resist the temptation to move to find relief. Resist the urge to relax. Just sink into it. That alone can diminish the feeling, but do whatever brings you to a stiller point where you don't need to move. You start by disconnecting from the movement cues of your body, from the sensory reactions, from the reality of sensations.

I am going to teach you a trick, not sleight of hand but sleight of mind, and, like stage magic, it's all about where you look and what you see. Now, this doesn't happen in your normal state of mind. Your normal state of mind is the one pinned down by pain, so, like an escape artist, you must undergo some transformation.

You might call this self-hypnosis, but I won't bother. I just call it trance. This is something you've done a thousand times unintentionally, so why give it a mysterious name? We're just going to take it a little farther, focus it a little sharper, and apply it toward a new end, though even that may not be true. People who know how to manage pain already know these tricks, and, as I have said, pain is with us always to varying degrees.

Now trance is not sleep, and that's not where we're going directly. Trance is a state of inner focus in which you use your mind to create a reality that has a life of it's own. We're aiming at separateness, as in that separateness is the space for novelty and power. Trance is the entry point to such a state.

Entrance

By this time you are familiar with the relaxed state, and it's important that you've developed that familiarity. It gets easier with practice and comes quickly. I assume only a paper screen separates you from your entranced state, and because this is so, I will quickly lead you there.

Sit or lie down, relaxed, present, and aware, and let that awareness roll down to cover you from head to foot. Take a deep breath, and let the air leak from your pores until a thin film of it surrounds you.

I'll count down from three to one, and you turn your outside in. I'll start at three for your relaxed state, here, now, present, and normal. When I say "two," draw yourself together like the drawstring at the top of a velvet bag. And when I say "one," loosen that drawstring, and pull the bag inside out, and find your awareness on the inside, looking out from the center of your chest. You just imagine it. Now go ahead.

Three, being relaxed, enshrouded in a warm awareness looking down on your body.

Two, drawn together, sucked up into your lungs on a full inhale.

And one, out and open, inside to outside, being inside yourself and looking out.

Leverage

Before you have always scanned your body's discomfort from the outside, but now I want you to scan it from the inside. You're no longer the doctor listening, poking, and palpating as we've been taught doctors do. Now you're the healer who travels on the inside, being the tissues, joints, circulation, and bowel that live inside you.

Go to a point that gives complaint. It could be an issue big or small, old or new, threat or worry, chronic or acute, a great trouble or a minor

The Path to Sleep

annoyance. Give this issue a shape, temperature, a color. Is it a fluid or a solid? A gas, like a cloud, or a plasma, like fire? An oil spill, a lick of flame, pointed like a star, broken glass, or grinding powder? If you poked it with a stick, what would it do? Jiggle, rebound, spread, envelop, or deform? Is it hot or cold, very hot or very cold, sharp, dull, slick, thick, sticky, clear or stained? Pick the description, and contemplate it such as it is, sitting there, just like you see it.

Go as close to it as you can. If you can, encircle it with your hands. If you can't, then sidle up next to it and detach it from you. Scrape it, shake it, blow it, break it. Let it fall into itself with gravity, rise with its own heat, pour as a liquid, or shift as a pile. Shovel it, toss it, kick it, detach, remove, and separate it. Now it sits there, and you sit here. Maybe it's angry or just indifferent, but you are here, and it is there.

Circumscribe your sensation. Without touching it, draw the glowing tip of your finger around it to weave a kind of light basket that does not touch it. Pull all the uncomfortable feelings into this basket, and weave this basket sealed, so it has no leaks. It need not be a thick or opaque basket, a membrane is enough, as thin as an egg yoke, translucent as a veil.

Make this container thicker. Make it first like an egg shell, thin and brittle. Then thicker, like an ostrich eggshell, which, if you didn't know, can deflect a hammer. Now a basketball, rubbery and hard. Heavier still, like a geode, crystal hard and hollow. Larger now, like a thick clay oven holding the heat, and barely warming on the outside.

Move this container out of your body. Move it slowly so that you feel it shifting. Change it as you need to, stretching, flattening, braced, banded, or buttressed. Whatever images flow through your mind, let them come and go, retaining the container and the feelings kept inside it. It doesn't need to be moved far, not yet, just outside you so that you can arrange and manipulate it. Bring it before you if you can, but if it remains attached, let it remain and just stretch yourself to address it, which might mean to face it or to face away from it.

Hold these feelings, your eyes closed and body relaxed. Breathe

Comfort

deeply... and hold your focus like a spotlight on a high-wire act. And this is not you on the high wire, and you don't need to be tense, and it's really more comfortable to let that tension be separate and you relaxed. Twice as relaxed now, twice as relaxed.

These sensations are encased, and they moved outside you, and they feel separate. Through this shell or casing there are controls, like wires to a radio tuner or the volume knob. The controls are on the outside, and the mechanism is on the inside, separate from you, so you can control the sensation, and you are not controlled by it.

Gently, gently move the tuning knob, and feel the sensation change its texture. It is pliable by its nature, this organic machine that produces strong messages and sensations in you. Explore how you can change the sensation's texture. Retune it sharp or soft, thick or thin, focused or diffused. Can you change the perception from what it is to something less bothersome, something dull or indifferent? Turn it into something you don't like, but you can live with, like country music, heavy metal, or Muzak. Something that you know how to tune out, like a nag, a billboard, or road noise.

There is a volume control, and you can turn this knob, too. Clockwise and the discomfort is louder, counterclockwise and it is softer. Turn it up a little louder, and then turn it down so that it's quiet, quieter, almost inaudible. Up, louder... Down, softer. Now turn it down as far as it goes, all the way to the left, and see if you can squelch, filter, or diminish the volume of this sensation to the level of background noise, or close to it.

Once you've collected, reconnected, diverted, and diminished the sensations you hold in this container, begin separating from the container itself. See it shrinking and moving away. See or feel yourself stepping away from it so that it sits intact but separate, like a hot garden grill, a whining wood chipper, or a smoking coal pit.

Removal

I have a case for you to put this in. My container is a sphere, pure white,

The Path to Sleep

half the size of a bathtub, and it opens like a clamshell. See your sensation as small enough to fit inside it. Shrink the clay oven so that it fits inside my container, and close it. Let them become smaller together and pull away from you. It's a floatable container, waterproof and airtight.

Imagine we are outside and there are trees. There is water and streams and a river the streams drain into. Imagine putting this container into a stream, and it is taken downhill. The container moves slowly, clumsy like a box, meandering on its way. It gets stuck, it stops, it starts again, it continues, and as it moves, it gets farther from you. As as it gets farther from you, you feel it less.

The stream meets the river. The container no longer stops. It bobs its way downstream at a constant pace, getting farther and farther away. And as it goes, so goes the echoes of the sensations in it, in your body, as you are now looking out from inside it. You can see that container, bobbing slowly like a lonely beach ball or an abandoned marshmallow. And the further it goes, the better you feel.

It may still be there, somewhere in your mind you may not be able to turn off, but you certainly can tune it out. Reduce its hum, heat, or pressure to an elsewhere sound, a hot sidewalk, or just another weight. And those, too, can be made lesser still, until there is no sound, or heat, or pressure, just a lot of noise, bothersome but elsewhere, there if you need it, but you decide, because now you can build walls around it, package it, seal it, and send it down the river.

This is just an exercise to contain and detach. To dis-encumber yourself from pain or sensation of any kind. This does not get you sleep, but it does get you comfort, because once you have reframed your discomfort, you don't need to keep extinguishing it. It is something else, and, as long as you are in that state, it will stay that way.

Find peace and quiet in that comfort, and with that space and peace of mind, you can begin to detach from other things: your body, your worries, tensions, and concerns. Once you can detach from how you feel, then you can detach from your story of who you must be. That will be a path to sleep, because in sleep you become someone else.

In sleep you become someone who sees through time, so the past and future connect. And you see across space so that far and near events are adjacent. Detach from space of separate locations and from time of before and after. Gain the fluidity to be at many times and places at once and no longer locked into one frame by an insistent sensation of the here and now.

And when we come back, know that the container of your sensations might not come back with you. Even though you may still be in the same condition, you will not tune yourself back into the state that you were in before. You can stay retuned or return to retuning whenever you like. Simply recreate the basket, container, the radio dials, the distance, and the detachment. Or maybe you won't have to, as you might not have reason to bring things back as they were.

Return

Returning back now on a count to three, back from being inside looking out, back to being drawn into the string bag of your awareness, and finally, back to inside in and outside out.

One, safe inside yourself, examining the working machine we've all so wondered about. Two, shaking out the sand and dirt, feeling clear, clean, and healthy.

And three, back here, eyes open, feeling rested, comfortable, and relaxed.

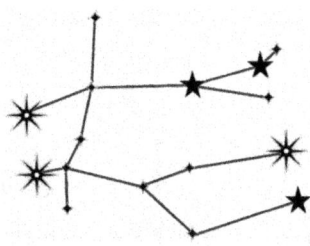

Hypnotic Session 14

Painless Joints

Audio file at: https://www.mindstrengthbalance.com/path-to-sleep-audio/

I assume you have a painful joint, or two, or more. Pick one and focus on it. I assume unless you move or put weight on it, this joint doesn't hurt too much. So let's start by taking the weight off and finding a comfortable place where you can rest this shoulder, knee, hip, or hand.

Consider the wall in front of you, and fix your gaze on a corner, a door, or edge. Fix your eyes on that spot. Imagine a line drawn between it and you, and let your eyes slide to a point in the middle, hanging in the air. Stare at the spot until you have a good sense of what's around you.

Close your eyes, and keep in mind what you were looking at. Open your eyes, and look again. Pay attention to the space around you. Close your eyes a second time, and imagine the room, not just in front but also behind and above you. Open your eyes halfway now, finding your place in the room, and close your eyes for the last time, feeling the room as it wraps around you in a wide circle, from left to right, far to the right, behind, and then to the far left and back around. Move further along that imaginary line until you are all the way inside you, at where that line is attached, somewhere at the back of your head.

Take a deep breath… letting it out slowly, going to that place of your relaxation. Focus on the structure and muscles in your shoulders… and relax them. Let them drop. Focus on the sense and space in your belly and at your waist. Take a breath, and feel those muscles relax… Focus on the big muscles in your thighs and calves. Take a breath, and feel those muscles relax as you get heavier in your seat.

Now we need to take your mind off this joint, to loosen your anxiety so that perception starts to dissolve, if only a little. Consider the egg… that's left in the frying pan. It sticks, and you can scrape it, and it will tear and flake, but it adheres. But then, isn't it amazing what water will do? Soaked for a moment in cold water, the crusted egg loosens and falls away.

If your joints are the frying pan, your anxiety is the egg, and I want you to run cool water over it, and let it start to come loose. And think of cleaning that frying pan, egg bits washed away so easily. And while you're at it, let that water run over your joint as well, and relax it.

Remember a time when you were active and uninjured. Remember this joint in particular. You never paid attention to it then, as it attended to your needs. Imagine what you could do then, and the full range of motion that was pleasant and easy. A simple motion, like walking, reaching, or tying a bow. Or simpler still: swiveling, bending, or turning a page. And in these things, a supporting feeling, and all of your focus on the action and what it brought. To turn to look, or lift, or follow, and these are things you still do.

I want you to sense the now-relaxed but perhaps swollen feeling in this joint. If you've lost it momentarily, then notice its absence, and then notice its presence. If you can, return to a sense absent of this feeling and then present again. Moving it in your mind, as it were, from foreground to background, to foreground, to background.

Gather back the feeling in this joint. It may be comfortable, or quiet, or not. See this joint in your mind's eye as separate from what's around it, as if it were a night light in the evening. Gather this light into a form around your joint so that the light it casts reflects the sensation you feel. Take a breath, and as you relax, imagine, feel, and become aware of all the sensation of this joint gathered into a warm glow.

There is another part of your muscular body that is strong and robust, a part that does not bother you and carries strength, resilience, and energy. This might be your biceps, your chest, your thighs, or your butt. Wherever it is, shift your attention to it, which you so rarely do, and appreciate that you rarely think of this muscle because it never complains, never needs your attention, and always supports you.

I want you to move the sensation of your joint into your strong muscle. I want you to take the injury that needs support and protection and give it that within the most able muscles of your body. And this is how you do that.

Feel the sensation of the joint, swathed in light. Feel the sensation of your strong muscle, always strong and resilient. Feel a path in your body from the joint to the muscle, and travel that path in your mind, moving through or around whatever bridge, obstacle, or conduit your imagination creates. This might appear as a sidewalk, a tunnel, a stream, the stem of a plant, or tissues and bones. Follow it in your mind from the joint, which hangs like a black seed, back down the stem of your body to the earth of your strong muscle.

Now imagine yourself able to carry the feeling of this joint, to shift it, settle, or move it. Imagine this feeling moving away from the joint, just the feeling now, the feeling that you've wrapped in light. Move this light container along the path you've imagined connects it to your muscle. Take your time, and stop now and then to breathe. And each breath is like putting down a heavy weight. It does not drop. It just settles, waiting for you to lift it, to go further.

Carry, move, slide, coax, or cajole the light-wrapped sensation all the way down to and into the open receiving muscle. Feel the sensation, be it discomfort or comfort, warm or cool, expanding or contracting, sharp or soft, and let it settle into the spacious area of your faithful muscle. The sensation is no longer in your joint, it's in another place, a place protected and well nourished, and there it can retire and remain.

Return up the path you've taken. There is a long drag mark, and you erase it. Sweep it away, and all along the path, restore yourself. Nothing to see here. Move along, move along. The new place is set, and movement in the old joint is felt in a new place. A safer place, one less vulnerable, less exposed.

What have you done here? What is it that you've tried to do? You are rewiring yourself, and why not? They are your wires. Funny no one told you, and you really can. And why **should** you? Because you might prefer it this way. So now your butt hurts to tie your shoes, and what good is that? Well, it's not so bad, and it's a start, and you can work with it, and you can do more than you'd suspect!

Settle now, and let the jumping nerves like jumpy children catch their breath. And you catch yours. Breathe deep and relax... Relax the joint... the path... the muscle... and your imagination. Return to the room around you, the space behind, beside, above, and before you. Remember that spot on the wall and the line you drew between it in your mind's eye. Stroke that line. Test it like a thread, and see yourself on it ice skating on a string.

Move all the way out, all the way to the door, corner, outlet, window, or wall. And when I count to three, open your eyes and be there, on that place, wherever or whatever it is, and take a deep breath of the presence of your surroundings.

One, back in the room, imagining the line that leads back outside yourself.

Two, following that line all the way to its end and cracking open your eyes.

And three, eyes fully open, coming back into the weight of yourself, and the air around your eyes, and your energy restoring your face, skin, muscles and bones. Feeling comfortable, clarified, focused, and rested.

The Path to Sleep

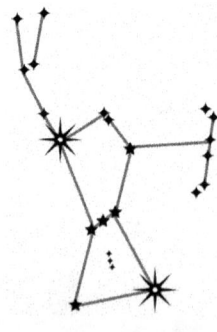

8 Accommodation

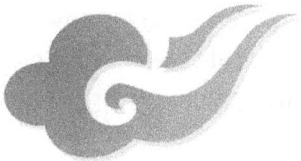

PUTTING SLEEP IN THE CONTEXT OF YOUR DAY.

More of Less

Think of your day as a loop and the events of the day happening within this loop. You sleep for part of that loop, and you're awake, more or less, for the remainder.

Each loop is different. At the same time, each day has many things in common with the next. The timing or beat of each day will follow a rhythm. The more you see the rhythm, the more you'll synchronize with changes and the less you'll feel the differences between each cycle. It's the "more of less" that is this chapter's topic.

I'm not talking about the diurnal rhythm, that clock cycle of getting up at seven, showered, dressed, and fed. Lunch at noon, dinner at seven, and to sleep by ten. That is a rhythm, and we will talk about that, but what I'm talking about here is what you expect, how you feel, and why you arrange your day the way you do, and in particular, whether this arrangement well accommodates your sleep.

In your daily cycle, there are things you feel you need to do, and there are things you feel whether you need to do them or not, and there are things you don't feel but should, because they affect what you do. Focus on what you need to do, become aware of what affects you, and accommodate these needs in such a way that allows the sleep you need and allows you to benefit from the sleep you get. That's what I'm talking about!

About the Day

You have sleep issues. They arise around sleep, and you think that by addressing them you will resolve them. Maybe, but let me suggest otherwise. Imagine you're piloting a large boat, and the bow is too high. You go to the bow, and you think that if you could lower it, the problem would be solved. But, in fact, the stern leaks water, and solving that problem will raise the stern, lower the bow, and level the boat. Your boat's problem is not where your attention has been drawn but in the other direction. So, too, with your sleep. Your problems may not stem from the patterns of your sleep but the way you organize the time that surrounds it.

Your job may annoy you, you may be agitated, and you may find yourself delayed in winding down to relax. You may feel lonely, spending social time out late, raising your energy levels. You may pour your late-night energy into your art, craft, or hobby. The point is not how you are or are not preparing for sleep, but what is happening throughout your day that you might think has nothing to do with sleep, but spills over into or steals you from sleep.

The exercises in the next series are designed not to lead you to sleep but to relief. Their focus is the virtues of calmness, soundness, control, and stability. These virtues may help you focus on sleep and reach that point where sleep is relevant, appropriate, helpful, and welcome.

Expand your view of your day, the phases of it, and your role in it. I suggest that whatever issues repeatedly arise for you during certain parts of your day—be that daytime or nighttime—be viewed as consequences, not symptoms. See these issues as consequences of how you organize your day or consequences of issues within of your day. See the emotional triggers that have rooted themselves in your day and whose consequences disregulate you later on.

The exercise "Winding Up" asks you to think about what you consider to be a symptom—be it agitation, enervation, or insomnia—instead as a consequence, so that a nighttime issue is also a daytime issue. This would be obvious if you drank coffee at 6 pm and then could not get to sleep at ten. It may be equally important but less obvious if you are stimulated at 6 pm and then can't settle later.

"Winding Up" focuses on putting yourself in a state, in this case a wound-up state or an awakened state. Whereas most of our guided visualizations are to relax and sedate you, this one aims to relax and elevate you. Your goal is to control your level of activation, stimulation, and arousal. You should be just as able to turn it up as to turn it down. After all, what kind of control do you really have if you can only go in one direction?

Some would say your undisciplined self is your emotional self and your intellect is the seat of your control. If this were so, then how often do you overrule your deepest feelings to act contrary to them? It is more subtle. Thoughts are neither stronger and righter than feelings, nor weaker and wronger than feelings. They are complementary, and they give a different perspective.

Thoughts are reasoned and create sequence; feelings are visceral and create consonance. They are suspicious colleagues, containers of different oppositions. One does not answer the other's questions. Conclusions do not resolve ambivalent feelings. Clear feelings do not provide reasoned clarity.

Drop the pretense that your thoughts control you or that you control yourself with your thoughts. See instead the contest between consonance and novelty, the attachment to pattern complemented by the desire for improvement. And if you do recognize this, then which in yourself do you experience as more powerful?

> *"A certain power to alter things indwells within the human soul ... emotionality of the human soul is the chief cause of all these things."*
> — Albertus Magnus (c. 1193 - 1280 AD), quoted by Carl G. Jung (2008). Synchronicity. In *Collected Works of C.G. Jung, Volume 8: Structure & Dynamics of the Psyche*. Sussex: Routledge.

This topic of accommodation is the largest of all our topics because it is the accommodation of almost everything, and this arises for us because we consider almost everything in sleep. What is being accommodated here is all complementaries. This includes the complement to wakefulness, which is sleep itself.

"Winding Down," the last exercise, is soporific, the complement to "Winding Up." It is an interesting experiment for you to notice if one enervates you more than the other sedates you. Can you engage these energies to move in whichever direction you choose? Or does focusing your attention on anything wake you up, or put you down? Those insights, by themselves, will offer you guidance.

Sleep is the rebalancing of all imbalances, which does not result in stasis or sedation, but in responsiveness, resonance, flexibility, and change. You sleep to restore yourself to engagement and to create accommodation for the whole of your day and, in truth, the whole of your life.

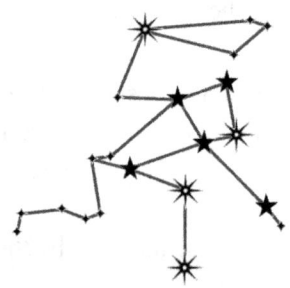

Hypnotic Session 15

Winding Up

Audio file at: https://www.mindstrengthbalance.com/path-to-sleep-audio/

This is a visualization for gaining focus, thought, and control. A visualization for the morning or any astringent alignment of limbs in motion, for no particular goal and every goal in general.

You want a sense of clarity and purpose that is a spotlight without needing anything **in** the spotlight. You are the projector, not the projection. You want to stop thinking as the actor and start thinking of yourself as the stage, to control the action—not by what you do, but what you focus on, highlight, or listen to. Do not aim to win the game but to control it. Control the game— not by how you play but by what you allow.

Sense needs nothing to think about. Being conscious doesn't depend on being conscious **of** anything. Being unconscious and trying to regain consciousness is the issue, and you don't do it by changing the script or the actors, because without consciousness, you don't have either. First, you need the house, the stage, and the lights.

I was unconscious once, and I fought it. I had no house, no stage, and no lights. I couldn't see, I couldn't feel my body, and I couldn't remember anything about me: who I was, where I was, or where I came from. I was perfectly lucid and self-conscious, but I was floating with nothing in nowhere. I kept trying to find, sense, or remember something but without success. Then I remembered the sound of a my flute, and as in recalling a dream, I found a foothold. From that I reassembled myself, or so it felt, until I had sense, vision, and memory.

It was a chemical unconsciousness, and perhaps it just wore off. Perhaps the lights would have come up anyway, but it's all that I can offer. If I didn't come back, I wouldn't be here to tell you.

The Spotlight

Focus is a state that is separate from what you focus on, but you do need something to focus on or else you can't know if you're doing it. You can't focus a microscope or a telescope looking at complete darkness. Yet once you have focus, it's entirely different from what you focusing on. The problem is this: If you're used to seeing things out of focus, then how do you know when you're in focus?

This problem plagued Galileo when he showed the moons of Jupiter through his new telescope. The image was focused, but the moons were not what people expected, so they didn't believe what they saw, and they didn't believe Galileo. And I'm sure he was all the more frustrated because you can see Jupiter's brightest moon without any telescope… a faint star but not the faintest, half a finger's width from the planet itself.

Having focus and having sight are different. And you really need both, because one without the other is meaningless. We'll talk about both, which may seem to make things harder, but it doesn't. It makes things easier, because now it makes sense. It becomes a science: You examine, and you confirm. And that's how you explore your state of consciousness to find out just how awake you really are when you wake up in the morning.

So here we're in a predicament. I want you to relax, but I don't want you to unfocus yourself to do it. I want you to relax but not go absent. I want you to relax, **and** I want you to focus.

Alert and Aware

What's a useful target to focus on? Let's focus on something that excites, stimulates, and arouses you. We're not going into forbidden territory because we need control, and finesse, and resolution, but of course we've already gone there, and I've already tweaked that bubble, dragged my nails across that surface. Just let it be like that, a loud report, over before you know it.

Something else, something invigorating. A walk on a chill morning or the dawn of a summer day. The rewound world has a tension, almost mechanical. I've felt it in the desert where there was no one to rewind it. The sun, the moon, the sky, the rising motion, moving sounds, chirping birds, and tapping beetles. It's ultrasonic and subsonic. Feel it through your skin. Feel it through your feet.

Step into a cable car, a street car, a subway car humming beneath you, all around you. Back to the wall, movement and direction, alert to people and machines—mind the gap, the step, the rail, the wires, the doors, the gears, the spark, the noise, the crowd, the plan, the time, the day. Movement with a bump, shudder, a veer, a tip, flex, and quick correction. Waking to focus on a train in fog, headlight boiling through blown and rising mist.

See the day casually wound like twine around a spool, a bin of oats to pour into your hands, a day's events to be picked out like clothes or breakfast. Where to set your eyes in a world that's waking up faster than what's in it? And over the near horizon, the next hill where your stomach sets, look for a rhythm where you'll feel comfortable.

Look to your body for the shifting of your moving, mental gears, upshifting from lazy to alert. Incipient motion of mind and the first creative thoughts of the day, somewhat muddled, still tongue tied. A foggy combination of grumpy, bumpy, maybe sad and happy, like the smell of buttered toast, breaking open to arousal, crispier at the edges. Listen to your feet.

The dreams are still there, always there, lingering behind the curtain, whispering to you. Your recollection is incidental, like your memory of exercise, socializing, or anything really. Oats, toast, cars, and stop lights. What's the situation, where to go and how to get there? What's routine, and what's your pleasure? What is your heart's calling? That is what sets your schedule.

Upshifting

Our thoughts often spin us around to move forward in reverse. Your search for focus needs something to focus on, but focus is itself a thing. Once focused, discard the object so you can focus elsewhere. A baby learning to

The Path to Sleep

grip must grip something. Once learned, they don't need your finger. But focus first, and then apply it. You learn to create the states that manifest results. This is how you gain control.

Where will you take the day, or will you let it take you? Set your clock, and set your cycle. Apportion a block of energy and ecstasy for your use only. And if you cannot place it, then store it inside you. It will keep... It will keep forever. Touch a shimmer of love for life and see it invisible, not seen by others but for being sensed, and you, too, may never see but sense it.

It is your directive to organize the positive of now, soon, and later into right order. Leave annoyances as rocks in rapids; they serve a purpose. You float over and past. You take a little scratching—not to your finish, rather a scratching with a soft brush on your back, your scalp, your legs.

There is a wind-up, and you enter like fast traffic, and you set the limit comfortable for yourself, and those around you acknowledge and accommodate. Create a landscape with the sweep of your hand, comfortable and pleasant as others see it. And there will be a winding-down later, over the near horizon after you're settled. Touch a shimmer of love in a still time and place, and you will reknow it and share it with certain others with whom you may be close or simply feel in the moment.

Within all of these cycles, there for moments passing, is the focus of the moment forming in the early of the day. The schedule accreting, condensing, collecting on the seed that is your sense of self, well known and appreciated.

Sense of purpose, known or not, sensed, and if not then find it, as it's essential, putting all in order, and needs no explanation. It's old, ancestral. You inherited it like a picture album of people you never knew but look familiar. Ghosts of your future whose silent hands build your day without your effort. Your hands and heart manage events better than your mind can, so let them.

Set it down, this task of priority and apportioning, and let it wrap around today's cycle, because at day's end will come sleep and—god willing and all in order—you'll put the day to bed and be ready to sleep. Then you'll return to the old faces whose whispering is quiet now, as now your talk is all that's audible. You'll give them full reign in your night time, in your dreaming, later, once the day is over. Now you have thinking to do in mindfulness. Appreciate the day.

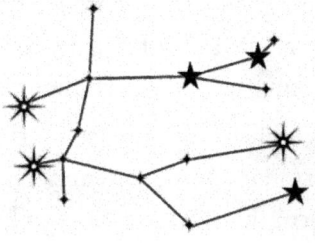

The Path to Sleep

Hypnotic Session 16

Winding Down

Audio file at: https://www.mindstrengthbalance.com/path-to-sleep-audio/

This exercise focuses on taking yourself out of the frame and unwinding your state to make space. Don't let go altogether. Keep your hands on the wheel. Just let off the gas. There are more thoughts we need and more turns to take. It may feel so familiar that you can follow this path in your sleep but not really. You can't. You couldn't sleep now if you wanted to, though you may want to. Have you thought about it? It's worth a thought, so stay on the wakeful road.

Going to sleep is not your target. That's short sighted. Your target is all of sleep: up to, into, and through 'till waking up and waking up **right**. And to wake up right is to wake up in right of mind.

Sleep is a ski jump you don't negotiate by just getting out of the gate any more than you would land an airplane by aiming to stop at touchdown. Prepare yourself in the evening by preparing yourself for morning.

What do you need to do now to be right of mind tomorrow? When you walk onto the tight rope, it's not with a mind of balance on your first step. It's with the mind for being in the middle. Did you know that? Can you imagine it? Walking a rope is all about the frequency of your attention and response, and that frequency changes and gets slower as you get farther out. And so it is with your mind at night.

Plan for the middle. Plan for the deepest part, the core of your experience. Plan for where you want to arrive, not for what's in front of you. This goes for everything: writing a sentence or life and death. And that's why sleep is so important. It's our chance to forge the big picture, our big dance, and what a blessing we have each night, a time to practice.

Organizing your day is a chess game between that part of yourself that strives for a shift to betterment and your symmetry-loving self. The first works to find a new pattern; the second works to keep the old one. These two differ in their objectives more than their strategy, as both can be reactive or proactive, receptive or aggressive. But the goal of betterment is to change what's wrong so that it might make right, while the goal of symmetry is to pattern itself to what's right so that it might keep it.

Let us play that game at the end of the day so that you may find the contest a more natural alternation, like breathing. Inhale and exhale. It's not a question of which is better. It's not a question of how to do more of one or less but how to make them work together.

Now there is no chessboard, of course, no black and white. And there is no taking turns—no score or checkmate—but sometimes it feels like it. Nevertheless, it's as useful to invoke what constrains you as to dispel it to release you. You see, relaxation is itself a figment: What unwinds one will rewind the other, so to relax your day, you must accommodate both.

This is what "relax" means as you wind down. What is your consonance or pattern, and what is your dissonance or novelty? Accommodate both, though you may feel it cannot be done, and logic may tell you so, convincingly. It can be done. There is a balance. Sit down with both, the logic and the emotion, the desire to start a movie at 10 pm and the reason not to, and let them play for and against each other. This is the game, and the goal is accepting the game and not the winning of it.

A desire to restore symmetry leads you to react at eight to issues unsettled.

Reason assails you with ambivalence at nine, for consideration.

Symmetry calls you to snack foods at ten, to find contentment.

Better judgment forces you to bed at eleven, in preparation.

Feelings counter by keeping you awake, battered by thoughts and patterns.

Maybe there is a truce, both give up, or a pill folds the game.

Yet once more, it is as your mother told you, or should have: "Play nice," "Be fair," "No one likes a sore loser." We think we outgrow these patterns, but we don't. It's still now, here, in yourself.

The Path to Sleep

Relaxation is not always relief. In fact it isn't usually. Relaxation is balance in alternation. How is there relaxation between growth and stasis, novelty and pattern, reason and intuition? There is none except in both together, in resonance.

Sit with yourself in the evening, the afternoon, morning, or night, and accept the game of opposites, the interfolding of freedom and constraint, volition and habit. You will not resolve it. Don't expect to. Want only to experience, perhaps to rearrange it, to place the pieces on the board as best represents this endless game. And this is what you do in sleep; this is what sleep is. It is when the spirits come and rearrange the pieces, setting the odds, setting up the dominos, the structures and constructions.

Sleep is not interfering with your problem-solving mind. It is re-normalizing the geography, re-leveling the playing field, remixing novelty and symmetry so that inspiration and regulation balance. Sleep repaints the lines and paints them differently each night. Sleep makes the space to play the game, and the more you support sleep, the better the game results.

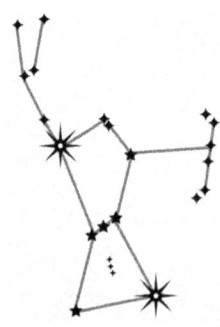

9   Habits

HOW TO BETTER ORGANIZE YOUR LIFE.

History

Our sleep patterns have changed radically with changes in culture. The most obvious change was precipitated by artificial light. Another influence of the modern era was the creation of cities, factories, and institutional work schedules. If you ever thought waking up to go to school or work was not natural, you're right.

Not as obvious but equally profound has been the development of beds, the bedroom, and beyond that, separate bedrooms for separate members of a family. Even having a private house—or during the early industrial revolution, any house at all—was not assured. None of these things are traditional.

Prior to the modern era:

"... it was commonplace for people to wake up and complete tasks; either to smoke a cigarette, use the restrooms, or even converse with neighbors. This break between the 'first sleep' and the second was time for thoughtful pondering on the earlier dreams of the night, even prayers, and were given great significance. In fact, these ruminations on early night sleep dreams lent themselves to the common superstition that dreams were somehow explanatory or predictive in and of themselves.

"The sleep that we are more familiar with, which became commonplace after the rise of the Industrial Age and contains no midnight breaks for pondering, suggests that we spend less time contemplating our consciousness, and therefore are at a

The Path to Sleep

disadvantage to the interrupted, segmented slumber which expanded the minds of humanity prior to our race to mechanize..."

"Prior to the nineteenth century the opinion of the time followed the Aristotelian belief that sleep originated in the abdomen as part of a digestive process called 'concoction,' and therefore wrote of sleep as a credit to physical vitality, lively spirits and increased longevity for it's role in the process..."

"... our modern, non segmented sleep ... has been a modern invention of the last two hundred years, rather than a scientific or cultural phenomenon of our ancestors. Our dreams, however unimportant in our western culture, have been consolidated in our seamless sleep. It is no small thing that while turning night into day with modern technology has increased our efficiency, it has also perhaps obstructed one of the oldest avenues of the human psyche for self awareness and personal growth. Perhaps the biggest loss, more than just the lack of hours, is to be 'disannulled of our first sleep, and cheated of our dreams and fantasies.'"

— Anonymously written, available at:
https://web.archive.org/web/20190721072937/https://historycooperative.org/sleeping-in-a-short-history-on-sleep-before-the-industrial-revolution/

Our modern daily rhythm, developed along lines of economy, class, and culture, has lead to a sleep pattern we consider "normal," a pattern that has us going to bed long after sunset, to sleep continuously in a climate controlled, air-tight enclosure on special furniture for equal blocks of time, to wake at a fixed time each morning. There is no historical evidence to support this pattern as natural or healthy.

The first lesson in improving your sleep is to regain control of your sleep cycle. If you can do this, then you will greatly improve the quality of your sleep.

The following topics address ways you can recover a natural definition of sleep as something you intentionally engage in after sunset, which you may enter and exit several times, and from which you wake up early, with much time for thought and reflection. Abandon your preconceptions. Explore your own definition of what your sleep needs to be.

Environment

Analog Clock

Place an analog clock (a clock with hands) in a location where you can easily see it while asleep. If it's visible, you'll see it at points during your sleep, though you will be unaware. Once you sleep well, you will no longer need an alarm.

Warm Extremities

Warm hands and feet facilitate falling asleep. This may be nothing more than a sign of relaxation because tension causes one's extremities to become cold. It also works in reverse: Warm your extremities, and you relax. Consider wearing socks to bed, maybe a hat, at least until you warm up.

Darkness is Good

Strong light anywhere is bad for sleep but certainly on your head as your brain senses light without your eyes. Especially disruptive are blue or yellow lights in the evening and night as your body associates these with the morning. If you have LEDs in your bedroom, cover them with pillows, cloth, or tape. Better yet, remove all electronic devices and their LEDs from your bedroom.

Stray light from outdoors can be annoying, especially truck, car, or street lights. I dislike cloth curtains and shades that create dust. Window shades often fail when the light source moves, such as the sun coming up. But, unless you live in a cave, it's important to have some means of controlling the amount of light in your bedroom. You might even try moving to a more cave-like place. It takes some getting used to, but it can be comfortable.

There are a variety of eye shades and sleep masks that may offer a better alternative, shutting out more light with less dust, effort, and greater effectiveness. They require some getting used to.

Get sunlight early in the morning after waking. Get as much sunlight as you can during the day.

Quiet is Good

Keep bad sound out. Let good sound in. Sound does not travel in a straight line, so it's hard to insulate yourself from it. Sound penetrates walls, and walls amplify low frequencies as that is their resonance. Sounds with enough energy will cause the walls to vibrate. Typical generators of strong low frequencies are motors and engines, which our houses are full of, or surrounded by.

I have a well pump five hundred feet deep in a well two hundred feet from my house. When that pump comes on in the dead of night, I hear it. When my heat comes on, I hear water flow through the pipes and the expansion of the pipes. Quieting my indoor heating is one of the reasons I run a woodstove as it's silent.

Higher frequencies seem more disruptive to sleep partly because one cannot help but to listen to voices, which activate your nervous system. Most music is designed to activate your nervous system. If music is audible, make it sedating.

Snoring, it is said, is a problem only to those it bothers. I snore, and I've slept in the same room as others who warned me they were intolerable, yet the snoring of others has never bothered me.

There are ear plugs. I have not used them. Sound machines, playing a variety of real and simulated sounds, can mask background noise to below threshold. Many interesting, long playing sounds are available over the Internet. Everything takes getting used to, and you can get used to noise as well if it is regular enough.

Cool is Good

A cool room, a warm bed. Close the doors, and open a window. Open them all. Make the bedroom cooler than what's comfortable to sit in. You fall asleep better if warm but you sleep better in a cool room. Your metabolism slows during the night, and the natural temperature at which you're comfortable will drop by a few degrees through the night.

At the same time that your body generates less heat, you are also less able to warm yourself if the environment gets too cold. If you leave a window open and your room temperature is not controlled, then your room may cool faster than you do, and you might need more insulation. Put an extra blanket at the foot of your bed. However, as I now will mention, with a better blanket you won't need to.

Insulation

Not all blankets are the same. Natural insulators are especially good: rayon, silk, wool, and down. Get a good quilt for even, rapid heat. The thing that makes great insulators great is how they adjust to your need for heat. They not only insulate better, but they remain comfortable over a wider range. This means that a high quality blanket will keep you comfortable even as the temperature changes. The old joke "How does a thermos know to keep cold things cold and hot things hot?" applies to great blankets. How do they keep you warm when it's cool and cool when it's warm?

The best quilts are made of down or wool. Down comes in many qualities and is often cut with feathers. Down's insulating ability is measured in the loft of the down and its quality in the percentage of feathers mixed in. Avoid feathers. How a quilt is stitched makes an essential difference. Baffle-box construction is what you want, and few have it. Know what you're getting.

Wool is rough, itchy, and greatly underappreciated. We joyously threw away our wool garments when good synthetic pile became available, but as blankets, wool remains better. It is uncomfortable against your skin, but enclosed inside a tightly woven cover I find it makes a better blanket than even goose down. For the best woolens, I turn to Scotland or New Zealand.

Natural materials are best as covers and insulators, but they can degrade. Enclose your quilts, throws, knits, and bolsters in tightly woven cotton covers to contain the dust. Shake them out, air, brush, and clean them at least annually.

Fresh, Moist Air is Good

Avoid dry air. Avoid sleeping in air-conditioned air. Dry air impedes natural mucus production essential for healing and protecting against pathogens. Dry air quickly dehydrates your entire body, taxing your whole metabolism. Consider a humidifier in dry climates, to allow for easier and healthier respiration. If you sleep with moving, fresh air, you will have solved this problem.

Bedding

Invest in quality cotton, silk, or rayon sheets. Try two blankets for two people, overlapped and independent.

Invest in a comfortable, firm to hard mattress. Firm mattresses makes it easier to move, as night movement is important and aids in maintaining posture. Soft mattresses deform, preventing motion and distorting posture. Yes, you do get exercise during sleep, mostly strengthening your back.

Your skin needs to breathe, and synthetic materials breathe poorly. In addition to ventilation above, you need ventilation below. Invest in a good mattress pad. Do not sleep directly on foam, rubber, or plastic. And over the years, all insulation gets compressed, loses its loft and ability to ventilate, and needs to be replaced.

Keep bedding clean to cut down on irritants to skin and lungs such as dust, hair, dander, and oils. Avoid artificial substances in clothes and bedclothes, including polyester sheets, pajamas, and electric blankets. Electric for pre-warming is OK, but don't sleep under them, on or off. Use high quality washing soaps to rid bedclothes of residual detergents.

Electricity

Keep electronics out of the bedroom. Remove plug-in electric clocks and appliances near your bedside and use mechanical or battery powered devices instead.

Keep electric fields out of the bedroom, fields generated by motors, condensers, and transformers in other rooms and outside the building. Turn off cell phones and Wi-Fi at night. Avoid cordless phones in the bedroom and use phones with hardwired connections. If you use portables in the bedroom, place them as far away from your head as possible.

Your walls are full of wires. Your dimmer switches have transformers called rheostats, and fluorescent lights have transformers called ballasts. Transformers, like motors, generate wide bands of electric noise, some of which operate at frequencies that may disrupt metabolic function. This is similar to the reason you're told to turn off electronic devices in airplanes. The airplane has its own electronic devices that are disrupted by what you bring along, and the same is true of your body.

Grounding

There is something called "grounding," which I feel has a positive effect. It is reputed to affect everyone, but I have evidence only from myself. It involves sleeping on a conducting bed sheet connected to the lower voltage of the Earth. The connection should be direct: a wire that runs from the bed sheet to a metal stake buried in the soil. To be conducting, the bed sheet must be woven to include threads of silver or copper.

Grounding requires you to run a wire through the wall or out your window to the exterior of your house. Silver-threaded cloth is expensive, so use a two-foot band that lays over your cotton sheet to make direct contact with your feet. Kits can be purchased for under two hundred dollars.

The theory is simple, plausible, and straightforward. You can find it with some research, so I won't repeat it here. The claim is the body's natural polarity is fortified by the lower voltage of the Earth, an effect we evolved to rely on but is now denied to us in our electrically insulated world.

The purported result is generally better health and healing, and it is my perception that I will often awake with a vibrating and energized sensation in my hands and feet. But among my small family, only I have this sensation, though I believe others would report it, too, if they were sensitive.

I don't know how this might affect your sleep. My suspicion is that it provides for me a strong connection with my body. Through that connection, my sleep seems more directed, my dreams more organized, and I awake with a greater sense of stability.

Nature

Get as much fresh air as possible. Ideally, sleep with windows open to bring in good air. We joke that fish are unaware they live in water, but how aware are you of the air you breathe?

Attend to the quality of your air. Many household materials release toxic gases: carpeting, furniture, upholstery, manufactured wood, adhesives, plastics, cleansers, foams, and paints. There are naturally occurring toxins like radon from the earth and carbon dioxide from boilers, furnaces, wood stoves, and gas heaters. There are irritants like dander from pets, dirt particles, pollen, and dust. Do you expect to sleep well in these environments?

Sleeping in Fresh Air

Sleeping porches were popular at the turn of the twentieth century. They fell out of use with the advent of electric fans and air conditioners. At the time, health professionals advocated sleeping outdoors as a way to bolster the immune system.

> "Researchers found that a week of winter camping reset the body's 'clock' to be more in tune with nature's light-and-dark cycle. The result was longer sleep... The study also highlights how modern living—so heavily dependant on artificial light—may thwart our sleep.
>
> "Saliva samples showed that levels of the 'sleep hormone' melatonin shifted compared with a typical week at home. Melatonin levels started to rise around sunset, and the campers' 'biological night' kicked in about two hours earlier. Accordingly, the campers turned in much earlier than their usual midnight bedtime at home. They also woke up earlier, closer to sunrise."
>
> — Amy Norton (2018, February 2). Time outdoors may deliver better sleep. *HealthDay News*. Retrieved from http://www.upi.com/Health_News/2017/02/02/Time-outdoors-may-deliver-better-sleep/9321486062450/

If you have an enclosed porch, simply move your mattress. If you have a sleeping platform, you can do the same to sleep under the stars. You do not need a tent unless it rains. Bugs are out only at certain times, and each bug tends to have its own time. You do not need bug protection unless the bugs are out when you are. There are bug nets.

Sleeping Outdoors

> "Do the stars rain down an influence, or do we share some thrill of mother earth below our resting bodies?"
>
> —Robert Louis Stevenson, novelist (1850 - 1894)
>
> "In dwelling, live close to the ground."
>
> —Lao Tzu, philosopher, sixth century BCE

If you want to sleep on the ground or away from a house then use a portable mattress, such as a foam-filled, air-sealed camping mattress. These are narrow but firm, light, well insulated, and they do not cause you to bounce in the annoying manner of air mattresses.

There are certain precautions to take concerning sleeping out of doors. The first is that the temperature can vary tremendously, so consult a weather forecast and ensure your insulation is sufficient. The second is that your sleep will likely be repeatedly interrupted, so allow yourself more time. You will also find that your rhythms will be dictated by whatever rhythms prevail out of doors.

There are also animals, and some are big, but even small ones can be scary. Remember Alfred Hitchcock's *The Birds*? We were seriously terrorized by parrots in New Zealand. They are no joke. Don't sleep near food or package remnants that smell like food. I'll say no more, but if you are so inclined, know your environment.

The primary rhythm will be the sun, but other rhythms will be the sounds of birds, mammals, and insects. You will be affected by changes in wind, air temperature, and humidity. These interruptions are not negative. In fact they are beautiful and amazing, but they can be a surprise, and you will need to change your indoor sleep patterns to accommodate them.

There are many benefits to sleeping out of doors, most of which appear to be poorly understood or under appreciated. Here are a few:

- The air is healthful and invigorating, cleaner, oxygen rich, humid, and well scented.
- The higher voltage on the ground leads to a charge that's absorbed by your body, helping to restore your body's natural polarity, an active aspect of health and healing.
- You are away from man-made electric fields, and you are in the presence of the natural fields of the soil, grasses, shrubs, and trees.
- Exposure to natural light sets your body's circadian rhythm and fortifies your body's hormonal regulation and synchronization.
- The frequent arousals you experience improve dream recollection and the natural cycles of sleep and wakefulness that prevailed before our modern industrial world.

As an alpinist, I had to sleep in some uncomfortable places. Once benighted on a high glacier with no warm gear at all, we carefully apportioned equal coils of rope between us as our only insulation, shivering in a huddle until there was light enough to go on. On another stormy night, sliding into the frozen bowels of a collapsed mountain hut, my partner Charlie Fowler famously said, "I can sleep anywhere. Once I'm asleep, I'm out." I've often wondered if there was logic in that.

Plants

Place plants in the bedroom. Plants filter, purify, and oxygenate the air. The soil of a water-loving plant is a natural humidifier. Tropical plants require moisture and have evolved to operate in low-light conditions. Plants are also sensitive to and exert some control over the electric fields in their environment.

Not all plants are equally effective at air filtration. See the list of effective air filtering plants in the appendix.

Schedule

Alarm Clocks

Set an alarm to go to bed if you need a reminder, but good habits will make it unnecessary. If you do use an alarm to wake, use the snooze for time to think and drift but not to doze or attempt to sleep.

Powering Down

Power down an hour before bedtime. Engage in different sleep-promoting activities. In addition to moving yourself into the rhythms of sleep, this will help you in going to bed at the scheduled time.

Maintain a Schedule

Develop and maintain a schedule. Habits are strong components to our schedule, and certain habits trigger subsequent actions. Brushing your teeth can be a trigger for retiring to bed, so each night after you brush your teeth you are psychologically ready to cease other activities and focus on moving into the bedroom. It could be a cup of tea or period of meditation. Let a habit lead to a rhythm, as the only difference is in the timing.

Naps

Keep naps short (half an hour or less) if necessary to remain wakeful and if helpful to retain equilibrium. I nap sitting up with the rule that if I'm tired enough, I'll sleep, and if my chair is sufficiently uncomfortable, I will wake up before too long. This seems to work.

Older people seem to have mastered the art of napping. A senior physics professor of mine, John Wheeler, took his naps sitting in the front row of the weekly visiting lecturer, yet he never missed a cue.

Sleep in the Bedroom

Use the bedroom, or the bed, only for sleeping or related activities: sex, naps, sleep, and so forth. Don't read in bed unless reading puts you to sleep. Don't use the bedroom for social activities or as a general play room. Kid's bedrooms are an exception as this is their only private space, but even then there is a benefit to routine.

Develop the mental association between your bed, bedroom, and sleep. If you cannot get to sleep or wake up during the night and cannot return to sleep, exit the bedroom. Do not allow yourself to project negative associations of restlessness, insomnia, and frustration onto your bed or bedroom. Take those frustrations elsewhere. Preserve an almost ritual association between the bed and restful sleep.

Develop Sleep-Support Locations

If you cannot fall asleep in bed, get out of bed. Engage in whatever activities seem to be on your mind. Engage in them fully and mindfully. After you get up, do something that addresses your discomfort. Don't do nothing unless that is part of a process of making space and self-exploration. Don't distract yourself with reading, movies, or television; engage what's creating the problem.

Make a comfortable place for yourself outside your bed or bedroom. Make it a place where you are both comfortable and can engage in relaxing activities. In that other comfortable place, make an effort to list and to explore, by speaking or writing if necessary, those issues that prevent your mind from engaging in the relaxation and expansion that precedes sleep.

If you wake in the middle of the night and cannot get back to sleep, stop struggling. Do not toss and turn, waiting without success. Exit the bedroom, and engage what's on your mind by asking yourself, "What is it that I can do at this time in the morning, or night, that I cannot or do not do at other times of the day?" The answer could be to take a walk or reflect on certain thoughts.

This may be the only time you wake up in this state, which might be worried, agitated, or anxious. You may need to make time to engage this issue.

Make a Deal

If that's the case, then broker a deal with yourself that you will devote a different time of your day, a time that is not disruptive of your sleep schedule, such as during the evening to address these issues. Commit yourself to exploring these issues repeatedly at this other time. Fulfill your promise to yourself so that you will no longer need to wake up in the night in order to consider these issues.

Eating and Drinking

Alcohol, Drugs, and Medicines

While red wine makes you sleepy, alcohol before bed wears off badly to dysregulate your sleep. Avoid alcohol before sleep. Drugs disrupt your metabolism and throw off your schedule. If you're taking sleep-disturbing drugs, fix that too.

Sleeping pills containing pharmaceuticals are disruptive because they're designed, like heavy artillery, to overcome resistance. The downside is their effect on the remainder of your sleep cycle and the up-cycle of your waking day. Some sleeping pills contain only naturally occurring ingredients, such as leading over-the-counter, brands. These may be less disruptive.

Of the many herbal sleep aids the most common are teas and tinctures. Sleepy-time teas contain chamomile flower and valerian root, among other herbs with calming properties. Chamomile can also be taken as an essential oil applied to your skin. Alcohol-based valerian root tincture can be taken by the dropperfull. Both sedatives are gentle enough for children but be aware these are true medicinals. Be cautious in finding a dosage that's right for you.

Water

Drink water before going to bed. It is better to have to get up to pee than to spend the night dehydrated. And when you do wake up to pee, drink another glass of water, which will further hydrate you, and help rouse you in the morning.

Food

Avoid heavy meals before bedtime. Avoid meals of high-fat foods that tax your digestion and spend a long time sitting in your stomach. They spend a long time in the rest of your digestive system, too. Some foods are specifically soporific, turkey being commonly cited. The key ingredient is tryptophan, a precursor to sleep-promoting serotonin. This is also the key factor in warm milk. Anything that slows our metabolism can have a soporific effect.

Serotonin production is helped by combining high tryptophan proteins, like turkey, eggs, or dairy, with the carbohydrates of any starch, such as wheat, potato, corn, or rice. Cherries and their juice are one of a few natural sources of melatonin, your body's sleep-triggering hormone. The high magnesium content of dark leafy greens appears to stabilize and extend sleep.

Prebiotics are foods that don't feed you but support your intestinal flora. These foods sit well before sleep because they don't require intestinal attention or alter your metabolism. Prebiotics are mostly roughage, raw vegetables, and fiber. As with most decisions, follow a combination of what your mind suggests and your body approves.

Junk

Manage your eating schedule toward late afternoon rather than late at night. Fats and oils turn off your hunger cravings, so it takes less of richer foods to satiate you. Avoid junk foods with stimulants and toxins, which describes most junk foods. Avoid sugars. If you're tempted, it is better to eat yogurt than ice cream, tortilla over Dorito® chips, and fruit rather than candy.

If you must have something sweet, use honey. Honey is half glucose, and glucose bypasses your digestive system to be absorbed directly. The other half of honey's sweetener is fructose, a fruit sugar, which must be digested and awakens your liver and a population of digestive organisms. Make your own chocolates with cocoa powder, butter, cream, and honey.

Body and Behavior

Learn to cease using an alarm clock as its use is a demonstration that you are not ready to wake at the time you need to. Learning this will come with better sleep.

Entrain to body rhythms: heart, lungs, stomach, and colon. Look for the rhythms in how you think and act. Explore your different body rhythms and see which are most somnolent.

Develop the skill of relaxing your muscles through visualization and guided imagery. Listen to the "Release" exercise from Chapter 5, the "Absence" exercise from Chapter 6. Take a hot bath to warm extremities and release tense muscles.

If you cannot sleep, at first or later, then get out of bed and write or read. Be mindful of what issues arise, and focus on lowering your metabolism. Avoid mindless activities that don't release you.

Heal Yourself

Apply self-massage by rubbing your limbs, both to relax and to increase circulation. Knead sore muscles, and apply healing attention and intention to injured or stressed tissues, even using your hands over and around injuries to warm, focus, and infuse them.

Your hands have a different electric charge from the rest of your body. They can be made warmer, and Reiki practitioners claim them energetic. Place and move your hands over key areas: genitals, lower gut, upper gut, lungs, heart, neck, and head. These chakra, nerve bundles, and gland locations are active in sleep and often chronically dysregulated during the day. Attending to the feelings in and around them allows the body to recalibrate and relax toward its natural rhythm.

The soles of your feet carry energies. Massage them. Place and move them over your lower limbs: soles together, against your calves, or folded behind your knees. Attend to the feelings in these places and those evoked by these postures in order to entrain to your body's somnolence.

Body Postures

Explore body postures that facilitate your connection with falling asleep. The anthropologist Felicitas Goodman studied trance states depicted in traditional and ancient art and noticed similar body postures. She concluded that these postures affect a person's experience and enhance your state of mind. More information can be found at these web sites:

http://www.cuyamungueinstitute.com/

https://neuroanthropology.net/2008/07/06/get-into-trance-felicitas-goodman/

Develop your own set of body postures that you can assume in bed, or before going to bed, in order to better develop the connection between your thinking and sleeping mind and your body. You might think of this as pre-sleep yoga or simply as a routine for relaxation.

Getting Exercise

Exercise regularly, preferably at times of high energy. Engage in easy exercise before bed. Avoid strenuous exercise within the period when you're unwinding your metabolism.

Ritual and Ceremony

Think about the coming day before you go to bed, and then think about how you'll shape the day while you're asleep. Imagine that going to sleep is praying and that sleeping is having your prayer answered. The ceremony of sleeping and the ritual of going to sleep focuses on connecting the intention of the later with rewards for the former.

Think of your bed as an unofficial church, and you enter it as part of the ritual. If you're not religious, then consider it a laboratory and sleep your experiment. In either case, you want to direct yourself toward an outcome that is more than just sleep. This outcome is a message, observation, or insight that you've created.

Make it official. Create an altar at your bedside, and assemble that altar from objects that are significant. If you focus on your parents, children, or spouse, then gather objects of theirs or that remind you of them. If your issue is your age or health, then assemble objects representing what you now want to do or objects from past times with which you want to reconnect.

Create a ritual that involves words, images, objects, and actions, all for the purpose of connecting ideas together in a way that will persist in your imagination. Strengthen the bonds between you, these objects, and your goal. You remember these, at many levels, in your sleep.

Hypnotic Session 17

A Schedule

Audio file at: https://www.mindstrengthbalance.com/path-to-sleep-audio/

This series of suggestions acts like stitches to bond the tapestry of your schedule, which you want to hold together as a foundation for good sleep. Receive these suggestions by first excusing the cold, actuarial receptionist of your conscious self. You must really want to consider this and give that person leave.

Create an afterwork situation when this receptionist has left for home so that these ideas drop like pebbles down a hole. That hole is you mind, and whatever strike or splash you hear is the sound of your own reflection, and you may never hear it as there may be no bottom to that cloud-filled well.

Find yourself a comfortable position. Carve out for yourself a space of thought-free time for the duration of these ideas and their suggestions.

Take three deep breaths, and with the first let the tensions in your jaw, mouth, tongue, and nose be extracted like the bubbles of a freshly opened soda, bubbling out, popping, to float away.

As the second breath fills your lungs, let its air be the tensions of your back, shoulders, and chest, and let the smoke of these be swept out by the exhale of an autumn breeze.

With the third, inhale the weight and bearing on your hips and thighs, filling as a sponge soaks up water. As you exhale, flush these out, like a hose washing away the suds, the vigilance of tension.

And with another breath, continue to relax down throughout your legs, filling your ankles and surrounding your feet with a thick warmth and light. And say and think to yourself, how warm, thick, and full you hands and feet are, how warm and full are your hands and feet.

Inhale… Exhale… Now you can see a threshold, or feel it, between here and the imaginary, except it's not. It is between being here, stated and acknowledged, and not here, unstated and yours alone. This is the place to settle to, relax into, to focus on not seeing but being there.

Go there now, and let a shudder of relaxation wave through you, shaking out the shoulders, spine, and bones, like someone shaking off a towel or flipping a rug to hang out on the line, in the mountains, in the sunshine, in the crisp air of earth and light.

Touch your finger to your lips, and say not a word. Don't tell me who you are, and don't give yourself your name. Reassure yourself you're taken care of and there's nothing to be concerned with. Relax again to feeling safe, protected, attended, and in touch with a deep sense of comfort.

Now let me tell you things that you have asked me to say to you. And if there is anything I say you did not ask for, then you won't hear it and you do not need to judge it. And what I do say that you did ask for, of course you need not remember who said it first, me or you, or who knew it more or better, or why, but just that I do believe it and offer it to you, if you'd like it… also.

The first is to have a schedule, a pattern, a cycle, to build a natural day around a deeper rhythm. It's the wireframe to your sculpture, a rhythm you feel as natural, comfortable, and attractive, and while you'll love and accept yourself when you need to disrupt it, those needs melt back into your natural rhythm, and your day-cycle does continue.

In this cycle there is a time—relax, open, and accepting—for concern with the meaning and self-knowing that you've been overlooking.

And a later time for judgment—relax, open, and accepting— for a task responsible, not forgiving, that you see best for yourself.

And another time for relief—relax, open, and accepting—that you can leave these things behind, to stop thinking, and controlling, and portraying as if you knew all along what you were doing.

Just a time to fall mouth open in whatever way you tumble, to sleep and simply drop your skin, your face, or hide, to be a vapor of your fullness, a sleeping time. Create space for it, and you like that, and it feels quite good.

The Path to Sleep

Now there are things that might disturb you—relax, open, and accepting—but beneath and through these, you cycle still.

In this you attract your schedule, and by the scent of your own blood, you will defend it, like a mother and her cubs. You are able to explore your feeling, how you need it, and you allow it… relax, open, and accepting.

There will be some testing and teasing by those who do upset you, for entertainment or adolescence, and that's alright because you regain your path, your schedule bobbing up, self-righting as a buoy.

There are cycles that you know of, cycles you wouldn't dare think to stop, no matter what you told yourself or others would suggest. They are your heartbeat and your breath, and I ask you to go further to the cycles of your attention and your hungers and your thirst, to the cycles of your stomach, your gut, and your emotions.

But still there's more, longer, slower, just as important, in your posture and your bones. And as your bones hold you up so, too, their cycle holds up your daytime. And as you would always guard them, so guard and live your whole day's cycle.

The cycle of your mornings, the unfolding of your afternoons, and the nodding of evening—let no one take them away. Put things in order after sunset for your nighttime and whomever will appear at the table you've reserved for the dreams you won't remember. Party of two, twelve, or twenty. No one likes to dine alone. Your allegiance is to them and not—as you might mistake—only to yourself, just your one and only.

Take a breath, and stop listening to my talking, and start paying attention to those of you in attendance. See those who are listening. Relax down twice. Simply drop your body, and hand the microphone to them. They have the voice you follow as I'm just reading from their script. And why you needed me in the first place is something worth your time to consider and… relax, open, and accepting. You might ponder on that, too.

Theirs is a cycle, a whole daytime, and see it from the outside. A stack of cards ordered by time and every one is you. Fan them out in your hands, from 12:01 back to midnight. It's your whole cycle, and if you have ignored it, then see it now. It fits like a key into a lock, and it turns one full cycle, and its tumblers click to open like a clock face. Behind is all your ticking, movement like a breath; a filling that cannot be done half-measured.

Your whole cycle, morning wake and morning moods, flowing to noon, stalking like a chicken, sliding into sunset like crocodiles down a mudbank, and ebbing into evening with a tired look on your face. This is your cycle, and you do it everyday, whether you're aware or indifferent, measured or oblivious. It is your chemistry.

So forget the words of all my talking, and remember only your first intention: to find your own balance and empower yourself to health. You only put me on the podium because, unlike the voices of your own, I follow your direction. And I've now read it back to you, and it's your turn to accept it. It was your idea in the first place to know the cycles that support you. And I'm not even really here but for the echo of understanding that I want you to take with you.

There, now I've told you. And now I'm free to go. You will create and command your own schedule, and you will hear and heal by your own inner clock. Everything is built of cycles, and they are as essential as transportation in this age of interaction. Let your connection with your world drive and enforce without distraction, the integrity of your commitment to the sleep-including cycles of your day.

Take three deep breaths, deep in the ocean of your awareness, breathing with the gills of your subconscious. With the first inhale, the bearing of your hips and thighs fill as a sponge that soaks with water. And as you exhale, fill these out, like a hose pooling, all comfort and contentment.

As the second breath fills your gills, extract the bubbles and fill your lungs with air, which, as they expand, touch your back, shoulders, and chest. Inhale for life and air and substance. Exhale feeling strong and crisp, deflating like a breeze.

With the third, now, fill sensation in your jaw, mouth, tongue, and nose. Bubbling up, here, there, past and present. Face flush, hands and feet, eyes

The Path to Sleep

open. Back and feeling great.

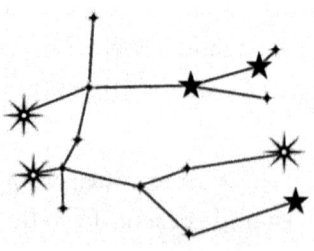

Hypnotic Session 18

Make a Deal

Audio file at: https://www.mindstrengthbalance.com/path-to-sleep-audio/

This is a visualization to explore your discontented experience of waking up in the middle of the night. We're calling it an exploration because we're accepting the idea that you're waking up for a reason. And it's not because of what you can't do but because there is something you should do, and you don't know what it is.

Start by moving out of your mind. You must do this because you will be asking these questions to parts of yourself that are not here now and are not even here when you awaken. You will only get answers if you ask the right people, and your normal waking self is not one of them.

Let yourself relax. Count yourself down. Five… Give yourself slack. Four… Let yourself slip. Three… Feel yourself settle down on a lower level. Two… Gather the things you'll need: a sense of fingers and toes. And one… to feel the surface and feet to travel down through it.

Open your inner eyes now—your third eye, your fourth eye—and see those vague outlines of the intermediate world where you can see what is behind things and perpendicular to them—just by knowing, not by looking.

Take a deep breath. Inhale… Exhale… And imagine that on your breath you carry your eyes, and ears… so that as you inhale… and then exhale… you see in front of you the experience of waking in that unready state in the middle of the night, half comfortable and enjoying the relief and half uncomfortable, agitated by a mosquito trapped somewhere in your mind.

And as you take the next breath—inhale… and exhale…—let this experience become a clear memory, sliding down the gauntlet of your arms and off your fingertips like water drops blown from a wind behind you. Blown to in front of you, and your arms are held out to it like a sleepwalker.

If your hands are palm down with a sense of distance, then turn them vertical, palms facing inward, embracing a sense of presence. If your hands are up, beseeching, holding, and supporting, then rotate them, palms faced together, to create space and separateness.

You are back in that time and space where you awake dissatisfied and upset... with seemingly nothing but actually something, something outside, something missing, something lost.

The discontent and disruption is not you. It's someone else, so picture them. Make them. Invite them, and assure them that you will hear them, see them, and respect them. It is likely that they won't believe you, so you must really mean it. You must get off your high horse, your authority, and be open to a story you may not have heard or may not want to.

What do they look like? It's alright. Give them any form. They will be glad you offered. So tired of your resistance they are that any effort on your part is welcome. Let them coalesce, like vapors into shreds and tatters into raiments. They are invisible people, so they wear face paint, and you see their hollows, and if you are truly humble, you will see their eyes.

Who are the people that come so late at night? Why have they found no other time or place? They are your children, and they need you. Perhaps, like the father never wed and uninformed, you never knew them or thought them someone else's memory. Did you know you live other people's lives? There are other children of yours besides the ones you have created, or will.

I say there is much that needs discovery, and I say I am not the one to say it. You are. And if the orphans at your door have come and waited in your morning hours, then you have to do more than stop sleeping in order to wake up. And clearly this is not the best of time or circumstance for meeting for either of you.

Take a snapshot of their eyes, and I ask you to bring your hands to hold them, to acknowledge that they do have substance and you do consider that you conceived them. You have heard parts of their message, and you would like to call it a disease, but you misrecognize your disquiet for a body illness, and it is not that. It is the ill figment of a dialog not yet heard somewhere in that body part that first awakens, perhaps your heart, your gut, your throat, or the sweat on your chest.

If you can do this, then you've acknowledged a responsibility, and you can tip your head to tell them that you care. If you've made first contact, not with a disease but an intelligence, and you can take this dialog to a realm that is proper, where they are not to be blown into bits of disenchantment but sheltered in the cotton of concern. Will you give them an appointment? Can you make a time of day?

Resolve to return to these images of body, mind, and memory on an even playing field. They only shatter the night image of your contentment because that is the only unguarded portal they can approach. Inform your guard to allow them, at a proper time of day, into a shaded time of welcome while the sun yet remains out. Resolve and promise to attend, to hear, to listen to voices that may have never spoken, and hear stories in the vibrations they have to tell.

Waking midnight discomfort is a message too weak to tag you, too small to hitchhike and stow away as a nightmare, but if you continue to deny it, they might find that strength one day. You don't need to let that happen, nor do you need to let it strike you in the muscle, bone, or joint.

Each day, or whenever, give yourself some time. And then accept the same discomfort you awake with in the night. And if you felt unhappy now, feel unhappy then. Sit with the hollow ghosts of your discomfort at a waking time of day, and resolve to simply listen to the braille beneath your fingers and the augers in the wind.

Perhaps it's not all so bad; I assure you, it is not. There is a healing at work here, and it's underneath some pressure. It needs space, and you need space, and in that space comes things you most likely do not recognize or mistake for who they're not. Welcome the stranger when you see them, if you see them, and you might not. So check the boundaries of your attention and the bottoms of your shoes.

Sit with them in the daytime, recalling every ounce of nighttime's disquiet. You must create all the memories and reflections that make midnight time so special and be as open and vulnerable as you have been then. In that space, when you rebuild it, sit and listen to the story your heart tells you. And in return, your heart will give you back your nighttime sleep. That is the deal you make, and follow through.

With that, let's return to this time, where we mean what we say and things fall into order and the disorder blows away and along with it, the shadows of your nighttime. They have another place now, an appointment. By giving them your attention at a time of day you value, they'll let you have back that nighttime bridge you need.

Back up. Return now, out of the cave of oracles. Put your personality back in order, like a stacked deck of cards, weighted dice that always come up snake eyes with, perhaps, a toothy smile. Back into this room and presence, counting up to five.

Inhale once from where you've gone to meet them, blowing like leaves.

Twice being where you fashioned it in your imagination.

Thrice to fold it back up, to stow it back on your shelf.

Four times to put your coat on, that personage that fits so well.

And five times, a brisk breath... feeling whole and fit to sleep better for the agreement.

Back here. Eyes open, once again.

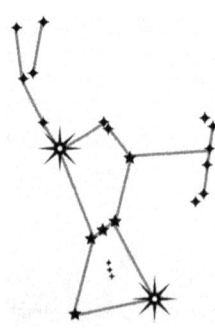

10 Dream Crafting 1: Outside of Dreams

DREAMS RECONCILE OUR PRECEPTIONS WITH OUR EMOTIONS.

What Do Dreams Have to Do With It?

We steer our lives according to what our superficial mind thinks, but we map our lives by what our authentic subconscious feels. Dreams are an opportunity to connect our conscious and subconscious minds, and we need that for guidance. They are oracular.

"An Oracle does not give you instructions as to what to do next, nor does it predict future events. An Oracle points your attention toward those hidden fears and motivations that will shape your future by their unfelt presence within each present moment."

— Martin Rayner, in Ralph Blum's *The Book of Runes*.

Reality for Practical Purposes

It is popular to believe that the past and future do not exist and that we live only in "The Now." I suggest the opposite: Only the past and future exist, and The Now does not exist as it can never be captured, examined, controlled, measured, or used by itself as the basis for anything.

The Now has always a duration whose measure is zero. The extent of what it contains can only be measured with reference to the past and future; its storage is infinitely thin.

If you have no memory of who you are and no idea of where you're going, then you are entirely helpless and without extension. Knowing everything only about the present is entirely of no use. This may not be true in the mathematically infinitesimal, but for our practical lives, it is.

Neuropsychology resolves this question using the notions of semantic and episodic memory. Think of semantic memory as a record of past events and episodic memory as your personal path through time. The semantic is your record of what's happened, and the episodic is your record of where you were in it. How could you be who you are without both?

That question is answered by the story of Clive Wearing, recalled here in a 2009 article by Suddendorf, Addis, and Corballis, titled "Mental Time Travel and The Shaping of the Human Mind":

> Clive Wearing is an English musician. As an acknowledged expert on early music, he had built up a musical career with the BBC when he was infected at the age of 46 with the herpes simplex virus. This effectively destroyed his hippocampus and left him profoundly amnesic. The nature of his amnesia illustrates the distinction between semantic memory, which is memory for enduring facts about the world, and episodic memory, which is a personal record of the past. Wearing's semantic memory is largely intact, as is his procedural memory. He retains a normal vocabulary, recognizes his wife and family, and can still play the piano and conduct a choir. His episodic memory, though, is profoundly impaired. He has sufficient short-term memory to be able to converse but quickly forgets about topics he spoke about or experienced just moments earlier. He is continually under the impression that he has just woken up, or recovered from being dead. His conscious experience is entirely of the present.

Clive Wearing remembers past history but has forgotten who he was and cannot form an image of who he will be. It is also possible to forget the details of the past but remember who you are. In either case you need a history. You must be able to recall a past and construct a future. If you can't, then you have neither.

I suggest that all that exists are the past, the future, and your location in them. The past, responsible for all that is now, and the future, the sum of all that could be. The Now is the boundary between the two, with no length at all. It is where you stand.

We do not experience the past and the future as similar. They represent two kinds of reality, one that has happened and the other that remains a network of potential. You think about the past differently from the future.

When you think of the past, you look for causes and their effects. You identify yourself as having traveled a path and being at some point now. Your paths may be many and complex, but they connect as only one through time. They can be traced, and the more you think about it, the more connections you find, though, relative to all you've traveled, you remember just a few.

This describes you up to a point. And that point is the limit of what you can remember, what you embody, and what has been recorded. Beyond that you're not really sure what happened. And when you think about it—though it's hard to think at the limits of all that you know—there is a lot you don't know.

As an exercise, explain to yourself why you feel how you feel about anything. I expect in less than one hundred words you will run out of things to say, and realize that you've hardly said anything! And what will happen then? You'll go off into memories and ideas tangential to the issue. And, after another one hundred words, that line of thinking will taper off, at which point there will be another.

By the time you're finished—and you never will be finished—you'll have created a rat's nest of bobbins and buttons, scraps and pictures, pieces of this and that that will amount to a comfortable concoction sounding like the ravings of a lunatic. And that, I suggest, is an accurate presentation of how you feel, why you feel, about anything.

This description of the past—all woven from reasonable ideas, each thread with its own logic—is a fabric that barely holds together. A crazy quilt. Take your hands off it and huge parts fall away.

Consider the future. How do you feel and what do you feel about any particular future path? Here you will create another story built on will power and what might be rather than what was or might have been, similar to your story of the past. In your future, all possibilities are real, though some are just more likely. Your future sprays into a mist of different opportunities at every turn, and you weigh them all to the extent that you can see them.

Your past and future stories are as different as can be. Birth is always in the past; death is always in the future. Nevertheless, both your past and future stories will be nests of reasonable ideas woven into a quilt of many directions. We are built of opposites, we think in opposites, and our stories are full of contradictions.

Which of these past stories is true in The Now, and which of these future stories will you follow going forward? You have to do something... right? Even doing nothing is doing something. Stay the course, or take an exit? Turn the page, or close the book. The scribe of time reaps every moment; opportunities come and go even if you're paralyzed.

Your stories are built from two kinds of pieces: short, reasonable threads and long, imaginative blocks. You stitch the two together and get a small tapestry, small because you don't have the time to create a huge concoction for every issue before you. And these tapestries, concoctions of sense and nonsense, are a collection of dreams.

Your dreams are a more accurate guide to and representation of who you are and where you're going than any one story could ever be. Being in connection with your dreams is important: Your dreams present to you the unseen elements of who you are.

The Importance of Illogical Thinking

I feel I must say things that sound metaphysical, as I suppose they are. Dreams take you beyond what you know, so have confidence in that territory. We need to talk about the process of learning what you don't know. Not the obvious task of combining two known things into their sum but finding understanding where previously none existed. That is the process of dreaming, and the more you embrace and indulge this, the more you will find welcome and solace in sleep.

A key to the universe is understanding the difference between the illogical and the irrational. The world is largely illogical, which means we don't know the logic on which it operates. There are as many kinds of logic as there are behaviors and relationships. Logic is about consequence, necessity, and prediction. Here our abilities are limited.

The difference between logical and rational is that logical presumes you know the logic that governs a thing's behavior, and there are an infinity of different logics, because there are an infinity of underlying principles. Rational behavior does not require you to know the reason. Saying there is a reason doesn't presume you know it. Saying the world is rational simply means things have a reason.

You are making a logical statement when you say all crows are black. You are asserting a rule. It is rational to say crows are black for a reason, and we may ultimately know what that reason is. But if, someday, a white crow shows your logic wrong, your reasoning remains intact. Before that day, you might have dream of multi-colored crows—illogical but not irrational.

Exploring beyond the known into the unknown is dreaming, and if you're comfortable doing this when you're awake, you'll likely be comfortable when you're asleep. Whether or not you are going to be comfortable with the issue will depend on what you are exploring. Thinking or dreaming about crows is not objectionable, but other topics may be. It pays to feel positive about where you're going.

And while you may not care, it is worth mentioning that both logic and reason allow for randomness. Things can be random and still have a reason. Logic and reason say nothing about whether or not the world is predictable. That's another story.

The point is, dreams are usually illogical but not irrational. Dreams are where you look for the logic that you don't yet see. You do this by rearranging things and events in illogical ways. Many of these relationships may not be true or only partly. Whatever the case, all dreams are a search for reason in an illogical world.

What a Dream Is

In an article titled "Envisioning the Future and Self-Regulation," psychologist Shelley E. Taylor speaks of creative visualization and says, "Like reality, a simulation involves a sequence of successive interdependent actions…"

But is reality a sequence of successive interdependent actions, or do we create the sequence and interdependence of the actions that affect us as time goes on? Our memories are mutable, and our reasoning changes. If our vision of reality changes, does reality change?

Dreams describe complete pictures not limited by grammar or syntax. Relationships presented in dreams are linked across space and time. Different dream events may be simultaneous. Separate places may be coincident. The story is presented to us as separated and sequential because that's what our rational minds best understand. That's how we remember.

Dreams present the simultaneous, the interrelated, and views of the whole before us. These views may be disjointed, as this is how we look at the world, or they may be the complete work. This wide view is often what we're trying to find in our rational, sequential mind through art, music, and literature.

Numerous artists, musicians, and authors, as well as scientists, have found inspiration in dreams and, on occasion, visions of fully formed solutions, melodies, and structures. I would not be surprised if many more people who find inspiration would credit their dreams if they were more practiced at remembering them. For more on dreams in art and science, see Dierdre Barrett's *The Committee of Sleep: How Artists, Scientists, and Athletes Use Their Dreams for Creative Problem-Solving—and How You Can Too*.

Holism is not a statement about dreams. It is a property of reality. An integrated reality is, by definition, a reality that does not separate things in space or time. We never see such an integrated reality in our waking state, but we can see this in dreams using our subconscious mind. The problem, then, is not remembering, controlling, or being lucid. The problem is understanding reality and the communication between the parts of our subconscious that have this understanding and the conscious parts that don't.

There is a long lineup of dream experts, and they have dozens of theories and interpretations. I won't bother you with them. Like a tin can, there are a hundred ways to open it, but all we want is what's inside. My aim is our empowerment, and my interest is in what there is to use.

I will give you one story, though, that comes from my physics background. In physics, there has always been conflict over which comes first, theory or experiment. Those who prefer experiment claim you cannot talk about what you have not yet seen, and those who prefer theory claim you cannot see what you do not know to look for. There is a kind of endless Punch-and-Judy, tit-for-tat between ridiculous extremes that wear each other down in sometimes interesting ways.

But here we're in the realm of dreams, and that leads us to psychology, if you want to be intellectual. Western psychology continues this cockfight in less redeeming ways. I find all psychological theories implausible for their lack of logically connected propositions, and for this reason, psychological experiment and its evidence is not compelling. It does not determine anything.

I find experiences with people most insightful, and here we can do away with theory. The fewer preconceived ideas I have, the better I hear and see. I am interested in direct experience and what we find that works for us.

Kinds of Dreams

I don't want to categorize dreams by content. I'm not interested in what I think your dream symbols mean. I'm inventing our own categories to mark the dream boundaries we travel across. What I'm setting out regarding dreams applies to waking reality, as well. These categories are not limited to kinds of dreams; they are ways to engage yourself. They apply obviously when we're awake where you're practiced in navigation. They are less obvious when you're dreaming, so these distinctions serve a greater purpose there.

Think of dreams as being of two types and then each of those types as having two subtypes. The first distinction is between reflecting and projecting dreams. The second distinction is between immersive and lucid dreams. I do not mean that all dreams can be so categorized but that every episode within each dream can be measured as to its place on these dimensions: more reflecting or more projecting, more immersive or more lucid.

This nomenclature is my own, and I present it in order to use it. I don't claim it's absolute, real, or even true. Today, I find it useful.

Reflecting

When a dream is reflecting, or reflective, you find yourself involved with familiar forces, times, events, intentions, actions, meanings, feelings, people, statements, situations, and levels of awareness. Unique and unusual events occur through your own eye in the first person. You recognize yourself and believe the experience to be real. Reflective dreams are an experience that brings novelty into what you think is real. Dreams are mostly reflective in character.

Novelty is a new awareness of something that has an emotional charge. What is often most real about a dream is how you feel about yourself. The dream may take place in a strange setting, presenting confusions and conundrums, but you feel and act in recognizable and familiar ways.

Reflective dreams rearrange things because you have encountered something in waking life that suggests you do so. Reflective dreams proceed plausibly but unpredictably. There is something new that's out of order in a world you want to see as logical or predictable. Your encounter with novelty is an exploration, a learning experience.

These dreams may leave you feeling satisfied and in control, or they may not. They are your effort to resolve conflicts. They are your effort to better resolve the instability in the world. Appreciating disorder strengthens your options, many that you may not yet see. We create our social worlds to set and enforce order, but this is never fully assured.

Reflective dreams release tension by allowing instinctive responses we repress in waking life. They let us integrate opportunities and abilities through the dream experience and indirectly through our interaction with dream characters who act out or inform us.

Projecting

In a projecting or projective dream, you find yourself outside yourself, feel as someone who is not yourself, or act in ways that seem foreign to your nature. A dream could be entirely a projection of a new persona, or it could transition to a projection or revert to being a reflection. Projective dreams confuse your reality by introducing a new self, a new goal, and a new set of limits. Projective dreams are an out-of-body experience where you're in a place unlike any you've ever been.

There is no sharp distinction between reflective and projective dreams. The distinction is more how you feel than where you are. In a reflective dream, you are bombarded by the familiar, while a projective dream creates a new perspective. Both may seem real to you at the time.

In a dream, I watched a middle-aged white guy in a short sleeve button-down shirt dance in place with his arms flailing. This scene turned into a large black woman sitting in a chair speaking to me. I don't know what the man was dancing about, and I didn't hear what the woman said. The message was in the context of the emotions of the moment. I didn't see myself directly. I was a watcher in this projecting dream. The result is not stored as memory. It's in the posture of my shoulders. What I invent now to explain the feeling in my body is the meaning of this dream.

Most dreams start as reflective and then complete or transition to another type. Recurring nightmares follow this pattern, struggling to find resolution in the familiar or else waking you up if you can't. You may move the dream to another context, retaining who you are and moving to a new location. In the context of lucid dreaming, which we'll consider later, this is described as remaining within the script, which is contrasted with breaking outside of it.

In non-lucid dreams, which are the large majority, you have little sense of authorship, so transitions just happen. Your authorship is set by your intent before you fall asleep.

Immersive

To be immersed is to believe what's happening is real. This is our normal waking and dreaming state. We don't question it, as strange as it may seem. We have faith that the universe is our container, and it operates without our attention. If something strange should happen, we figure it's just the way things are.

Evocation of the strange is something we reserve for fantasy, and sometimes we call it art. We indulge in it with regularity in movies and music, with happy or angry satisfaction. We distinguish this from what's real, but, with a moment's reflection, the two always dance together.

When deeply immersed, you are at the mercy of events, though you do have more control than a leaf floating in a stream, you may choose coffee or cappuccino, but can you decide when to take a break? Your control feels proportional to your preparation, as with a week's notice, you may set your time, but the limits are that of the web you're in, which—and you'd better face it—is a web you have created. Being immersed is being enmeshed. You consider your options in a reality that you take for granted.

When dreaming, you have a short memory and your thinking is short term. You're rarely planning for the next day as the dream's future is unpredictable. You don't know how to arrange it. In an immersive state of mind, your decisions are determined by your situation. This is how you want it; this is a projection of your desires. You want your reality to unfold comfortably and without your effort.

In real life, and as in dreaming, the immersive reality is not true. You are responsible for almost everything, and you are the one who maintains it. Others have created other lives, and they're not all that different from you. Their circumstances were and continue to be different, but with the broadest understanding, everything can be shaped. When you become aware, then you realize none of this has to be. That is the lucid state, and it is as unusual in dreaming as it is in waking reality.

Lucid

To lucid dream means to be in control and, at first, this distinction seems quite clear. Early, enthusiastic researchers thought lucidity was a separate state, but now it has been recognized as not so clear or separate. It's a matter of degree.

How do you know just how much "free will" you have in a world you've never before encountered and will never experience again? What if your "free will" is based on memories you had no hand in creating? And what is free will anyway, and is your memory real? You may "know" you're dreaming, but that doesn't explain what's going on. These questions don't plague you now, but if you've woken up five times, and each time find yourself still dreaming, you might start to wonder.

Lucidity exists on a spectrum. Psychologists might say, "Reality is a spectrum disorder." Dreams are similar to stage plays. There is an author, there is a theme, and there are actors, but it's never entirely clear which is which. Are you the dream's author or its actor? Are you playing a supporting role, or is the play about you? And if you feel free will such as to declare, "This is a dream!" did you extemporise that line or was it written in the script?

It's not all that important to answer these questions, but asking them makes the experience richer. It can help you see the new possibilities. By the time you're finished here, you'll see that many of the questions we cannot answer about our dream states we cannot answer about our awake states either.

The Dream Conversation

In most courses on dream work, this section would be called "How to Interpret

Your Dreams." I don't think that's useful, and I don't want to call it "dream interpretation" because this is not a laboratory. Dreaming is a two-way process, a conversation, and there is as much for you to say through dreaming as there is for you to hear.

In quantum mechanics, there is something called "the observer effect," which is a fancy way of saying that you can never be objective in your examination of something that you create. There really is no clear separation between the examination of your dreams and your creation of them.

That is not to say you cannot reflect on what you remember but rather that what you remember will change as a result of your reflection on it. There is no fixed anything about dreams, and you don't even want to go there. As you explore your dreams, or even just your feelings, if you lack a clear recall, then they will talk back to you, and they will tell you how to understand them.

You don't need a tourist's guide, and you don't need to speak "their language." Your dreams are your deeper self, and if you don't answer when they call, they'll leave you a message. Understanding the message is the issue, and for that you'll need to do some work. You are the bug under the microscope, not them. If you don't yet "get it," then keep trying. It's all about your being receptive, perceptive, ready, and accepting. When you've demonstrated enough promise and displayed enough intelligence, your inner mind will let you know what's going on.

The Unimportance of Remembering Dreams

Now, you might wonder if you have sufficient dream recall or if you dream at all. You should not be overly concerned. I never said dreams need to be remembered because, for the most part, they are forgotten. You may have a dozen dreams each night and remember none, or one occasionally. Dreams do not need to be remembered to be effective because their effect is not on your memory but on your character.

Dreams affect what you think, how you think, and how you feel—aspects of yourself always and immediately available. You don't have to "think" about how or what to think. This just happens. You don't have to remember the stories contained in your dreams, just as you don't need to remember the meaning of words. You just use them. Your dreams take, consider, attach, disassemble, and digest information. They integrate and rearrange the concordances and causalities of your thoughts and feelings and other such things that constitute who you are.

If you don't need to remember your dreams, why are we talking about them? Because they offer an opportunity for growth and a better life. And, while we generally don't remember our dreams, we benefit from working with them when we do.

What might it mean to work in order to effect something you can't recall? A sort of "pin the tail on the donkey" you never get to see. It's not really the dreams we're concerned with unless, like nightmares, they are a concern in and of themselves. We're concerned with how we think and feel.

Dreams are intermediate stages in the integration of events into our personality. If we can change ourselves by working with dreams indirectly, we accomplish what we set out to do. It may be all the easier to consider dreams as unconsciously as our digestion, to simply feed them, and they will do their work.

Remembering

I suspect you will begin to remember your dreams simply as a consequence of becoming familiar with the state of being "in between." I make no special effort to remember my dreams, but my normal efforts put me in closer touch with them than is usual for most people. On the other hand, dream recall does require some completion of your sleep cycle and improves with the quality of your sleep. Presumably, given the topics of this book, you have problems with sleep completion and quality. If dream recall will not improve your sleep by itself, then let dream recall be a goal for other reasons.

If you want to be proactive in dream recall, the prescription is simple and direct: Wake yourself while you're dreaming. This means you need to wake during one of your REM cycles, and these cycles become longer and more frequent as the night ends, extending to as long as forty minutes, separated by ten minutes of light non-dreaming sleep. During all these REM periods, it is presumed you're dreaming, yet all you're aiming to recall is just a bit of the last one.

If you're well slept, then waking up during the inter-REM periods is easier and less disturbing. Well-rested people who extend their mornings will also have a better sleep. Lacking the luxury of a leisurely morning, try using an alarm clock to wake yourself from a dream cycle. Personally, this does not appeal to me; it's too much like drawing blood, but it will cause you to remember dreams!

When waking from the alarm's disturbance, focus only on what you recall. Don't move or look around. Don't think about your day or any of your daily concerns. Dreams are fragile, and their traces are quickly lost. Write what you recall in a dream journal, either as an outline or in detail. If you have the time, wake yourself repeatedly throughout the morning to recall multiple dreams.

In my own work, I find more than an occasional dream to be a burden, like eating too much chocolate. I much prefer to fashion pre-sleep fantasies and then savor as many dream wisps as I remember.

As I say, I don't make a special effort to do this, but because I often sleep outdoors, I almost always wake up before dawn and move inside where I return to sleep. When I do recall my dreams, it's not because I made an effort to but because they feel important.

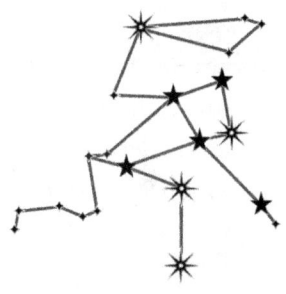

Hypnotic Session 19

Building a Dream

Audio file at: https://www.mindstrengthbalance.com/path-to-sleep-audio/

The boundary between being awake and asleep is not as sharp as people think. It's not air versus water but more air versus cloud, and in between there is fog, and drizzle, and mist. Your senses can lift off the ground; your sight can see what is somewhere else.

You are already preoccupied with what's in your mind's eye, and your senses are already planted in a world that is not here. You are already built into a vision you have created with such fervency you won't release it. You've got a mindset that is way too narrow. You've made it hard to get to sleep.

You stand stretched on tiptoes, straining to grab the sleep ring. There are steps you can build, a step stool to reach those higher shelves. Don't be a jerk. Learn to do it right before you sprain yourself!

First, don't stretch. Relax. Relax your body. Relax your mind. Are you comfortable now? Get comfortable. If you're on a bed or on a floor, in a reclining chair or sitting on a bench, find a pillow, straighten your spine, and let gravity kiss the backs of your legs or the bottoms of your feet.

Relax your nerves at the top of your scalp, your temples, forehead, and around the back of your head where your second eyes are. Close those radar eyes, and feel comfortable with what's behind you. Close your forward eyes, and feel comfortable with what's in front of you.

Let a host of tiny fairies massage the muscles of your face to relax your cheekbones, eye sockets, eyebrows, the hollows of your cheeks, the hinge of your jaw, and the gums of your teeth. As if these little people were cleaning lichen off Mount Rushmore, let them smooth down the bridge of your nose, relax your tongue, and separate your teeth so that they can scrub your bitting surfaces.

Dream Crafting 1: Outside of Dreams

Pull the pins that hold up your shoulders, and let them settle just a bit. Open the valve and let your breath exhale all the way so that your ribs settle down and you breathe from your stomach. Your arms relax and sink heavier, warmer... heavier... Grease your hip joints with the tingle of lubricant so you can feel them vital and unweighted all the way down your thighs and legs, in through your knees, and down to you ankles. Check the nerves on the bottoms of your feet. Can you feel your heels? Your arch? The sides of your feet? The balls of your feet? Can you feel your toes? Good. Let them tingle, feeling warm, feeling heavy.

Let me count down, and you focus on how wide, deep, and relaxing each number feels.

One hundred. Just starting and you're relaxed.

Ninety-nine. More deeply relaxed, more relaxed.

Ninety-eight. Calm, wide, warm, and relaxed.

Ninety-seven. Serene. Relax more deeply.

Ninety-six. Comfortable, quiet, dreamy, drowsy.

Ninety-five. Drifting, turning, rocking, releasing.

Ninety-four. All the way relaxed, just to be relaxed.

Ninety-three. All the air out, breathing deep and slow.

Good.

This is where we want to be. This is where we want to hold this conversation.

What do you do first when you lie down to sleep? Do you look at the clock, or look out the window? Drowsy eyes drifting from a television, at the blinking light on the ceiling. Or do you close your eyes to try to see nothing? Is this the send-off you give yourself?

You won't remember most of your dreams, but that doesn't mean you didn't set their theme. Imagine your dream actors opening their lunch to find another peanut butter sandwich, waking up to find themselves in the same neglected, dingy theater, to rail against the you, their landlord, with whom they can never get in touch.

You think you can loll, indifferent, and just collect the rent while your dream theaters decay? Every night you struggle to sleep, distracted. You create another crack in the foundation, a leak in your dream's roof.

Let me tell you how you should shove off into sleep's deep waters; you should do it right. You should first look deeply into the most beautiful and mysterious thing you can imagine. Something, or somewhere, that holds everything for you. And that place or thing is always available, if you can imagine it. Imagine it!

Place yourself somewhere else entirely, in the nighttime on a warm, sand beach, beneath a jewel-encrusted sky, enveloped in a deep armchair before a glowing fireplace, high on a mountain top above a wild and untamed landscape, wrapped in weavings and painted silks, surrounded by a community of family and children, swimming as a dolphin in a sea below two suns. What does it look like, feel like, sound like, smell like?

Smell is our oldest sense. Even bacteria have it. It is the chemistry of our surroundings. So what does the most beautiful and mysterious thing you can imagine smell like? What is the sense of its scent? Take this as your brain's deepest trigger, one that will take you right to this place for certain.

Is it somewhere you are, have been, have known, or could ever get to? For me it is the deep night sky because that's where I put it, and its scent is the open, clear air after a thunderstorm. It could be your home, the ocean, the city, or the curve of the earth, scents of cinnamon, hay, or salt water. This is where you want to be connected, which no one can take away. This is your creation.

Try this next time you turn off the lights and paint your perfect place. Say to yourself, and enunciate quite clearly, "Please connect me with the characters in my dreams tonight," and then just wait, like you're on hold, until something happens.

You may think it odd or quaint to expect an answer in speaking to yourself, but it is how we make connections all the time: rumination,

Dream Crafting 1: Outside of Dreams

supplication, introspection, affirmation, declamation, determination. We're always talking to ourselves. And if no one was listening, why would we ever bother?

Do you know where words came from in their written form? They were pictograms of life's meaning, objects imbued with spirit. "The Mystery" spoke through them, and it still does because The Mystery is still listening.

Now, what exactly happens, I cannot say. You could be shocked to hear a voice say, "Hello." Some images may just drift past in your mind. You may need to look and listen, and you may need to almost turn around to see. If you've not practiced this, the response may be fleeting, like a bad phone connection to a foreign country, but with practice, the connection gets better, and you will find your call put through.

More than likely, something will come to you. It usually does when you ask. You may not recognize these characters, and they may not recognize you're on the line. Hold on to those willing to be kept waiting, and pursue those who continue on their way, until you've got some characters variously costumed in your mind.

Speak to them as if at a briefing, audition, or rehearsal. Tell them what you'd most like to accomplish, and request that they help you. They respond to your heartfelt emotion, so let them know how you really feel. They are not just actors but emissaries. They perform in higher roles. They have an "in" with forces that make things happen, and if you convince them to present your case, a higher focus will put your true intention in the spotlight.

Please suggest to these agents the scene and the setting, even if it seems outside their natural form. They are shape shifters by their nature, and they have played many roles in your past dreams. Saints, monsters, heroes, and children, and they have connections with all the others. They can read your mind if you make the effort.

You have recalled a mysterious place of beauty. You have spoken of what you'd most like to do. You've gathered the attention of your agents and a scene in which this might take place. Combine these in your mind: a mystery, a goal, characters, a place. Hold these all together with a sense of duty to yourself and purpose, a meaningfulness that is not the least bit tired. Mate this with a deep relaxation, as if you have now done everything you can to make this happen.

Take a deep breath, and with your inhale, place yourself in your sense of mystery. With your exhale, blow pixie dust on the actors, their setting, and the theme. Do this right and they'll smile at your good intentions.

One good turn deserves another as every actor loves a good script. Create for them the opportunity to play a deep and meaningful role, and they'll reward you with the performance of your life. It's a performance they do a dozen times each night and roles in which they never tire. They can feed you energy that you never knew you had. When you focus on what really matters, your body answers the calling.

Let this become a mantra, a one-breath affirmation you can repeat. Deeply inhale the scents of mystery. Exhale the actors and the theme. With your fading breath, sink into the audience. And with the next inhale, repeat the mantra: that idea that's most important to you. Keep repeating this cycle as you fall asleep.

You know, it doesn't really matter if they perform your play or if you remember. The message is delivered whether or not you wake up for the performance. You have a dozen dreams each night, and you are lucky if you remember one. You are not even the intended audience. The show is put on for angels as it's they who shape the world. And don't be afraid of demons because they just twist the plot. Someone has to break the set, and they're always wearing black.

There are dark forces. I don't know their role. You cannot let fear stop you; most of it is not what you think. And the things we really need to be afraid of are things we really need to fix. There are dirty, dangerous jobs, but those tasks wouldn't be before you if you were not the special one to perform them.

We all look for heroes, and some part of you is one. There are certain things you didn't create that you are here to fix, regardless. Take on these tasks and reap the hero's true reward: to be spared the curse of credit and the blessing of making other people happy.

You have a mantra. Use it. Refine it. Explore it. It's better than any sleeping pill. It may not always be effective, but you can never overdose. It's a powerful elixir, a spell, a charm, a prayer. You create what you focus on, and so what if you don't know what's most important, you can still look for it. And if you do, you'll find it's like a good leather shoe. It softens as you wear it and becomes a second skin. It will carry you through field and stream, city and jungle, to the highest accomplishments and the deepest sleep.

Now I want to go to sleep. If you don't want to, then you can come back to your alert state. If you do want to sleep, then follow me forward as I continue with counting down.

Ninety-two. Relax.

Ninety-one. Calm, wide, warm.

Ninety. Serene, relaxed, open, aware.

Eighty-nine. Comfortable, quiet, dreamy, drowsy.

Eighty-eight. Drifting, floating, rocking, releasing.

Eighty-seven. All the way relaxed, just to be relaxed.

Eighty-six. All the air out, breathing deep and slow.

Eighty-five. Heartbeat slow and smooth. Center on your heart.

Eighty-four. Center on your breath. Inhale... Exhale...

Eighty-three... Deeply relaxed.

Eighty-two... Deeply relaxed.

Eighty-one... Done.

The Path to Sleep

Hypnotic Session 20

Transitions

Audio file at: https://www.mindstrengthbalance.com/path-to-sleep-audio/

Find a comfortable position with both feet on the floor. Take a breath. Inhale… Exhale… and place your two hands atop your chest. Place one higher at your collarbone so that the fingertips of that hand rest at the center of the bone, just under your chin.

Place the other hand lower, at the bottom of your sternum, so that the fingertips rest atop the bone at the center of your chest. Touch, rub, or press these places as you feel comfortable. You'll tap your fingers to focus your attention.

This exercise is about making time for yourself, a time in which you can leave open a channel between your declarative, demanding self—the self that accepts only what's real—and your imaginative, receptive self—the self that invents what's real. This will be a time between feeling who you are and who you could be. It's quite simple. All you need is the sense of both of these selves as allies and the commitment to give yourself some time.

Waking

There is a time between when you begin to wake and when you feel you are awake that is an in-between state. This is an important time, when you're between worlds. It is in this state, not just in the morning but anytime, that we access strength and balance and fuel our mental health.

In this time, you can consider the blocks your subconscious fashions in your dreamtime. You don't have to do anything, just allow the two worlds to mingle free from the interfering judgment of your daytime mind.

This time and times like these connect to your individuality and are key times in connecting with yourself. This morning wake-time is held in reverence in all contemplative traditions, a time of prayer, meditation, and reflection. We will explore the power that lies in this time, so I'll ask you to create it.

You want the space between dreamtime, which you may or may not remember, and the daytime, which you'll certainly forget. Go beyond the simple "being in touch" with memories and conversations to the deeper "being in touch" with how and why you feel.

Be in touch with direction and inclination, the kind of direction you associate with road signs, parts and meaning, emotional triggers, and auspicious events. Be inclined to span possibilities and reactions. Go beyond the simple questions of what, why, where, when, and how, and ask this of many feelings.

Go beyond a single pin-hole focus, and welcome the shifting, fluid texture of near- and far-term goals. You don't need detail or enumeration, just the questioning sniff of association and instinct. Stir ideas, not separate but brought together. Ask yourself directly, "What are the feelings I woke up with?" Listen to the answer you hear now.

Your memory is the barest of bones. What you recall is always clothed in the suggestions of your imagination. This isn't just memory. It's everything, as most of what you see, hear, taste, smell, and feel, you make up. The senses are just triggers. Memory is a shell and imagination the powder—the two parts of the ammunition of recollection.

Watching

Recall how it was when you woke up this morning, and imagine you are just waking up now. Recall an image from the night, last night, any night, or whatever comes in this moment. Watch your thought. Examine it. Consider your emotion. Sit with your feelings. Don't think too much. See or feel what comes first to your mind. This is the first idea, and that's what we'll call it: the first idea.

If your two hands are not on your chest, put them there. With one hand's fingertips on your collarbone, slowly tap together on that bone: TAP… TAP… TAP… And in alternation, tap the fingertips of your other hand on your sternum. Alternate: tap above, tap below, tap above, tap

The Path to Sleep

below. Tap in the cadence of my words in double-time with your heart beat: TAP, tap... TAP, tap... TAP, tap...

Just keep tapping gently, and I will tell you when to stop. It's just a way of triggering emotions from your body so that you can see them, like shaking apples from a tree. I want you to be open without expectation, just to watch yourself from the perspective of a thought.

As you're tapping, look forward beyond your feeling, and this can be in any way you take it, and how you take it won't matter because all these meanings are related. Explore the "more" of it and the less. What shakes, in this tapping, from beyond that feeling? And if nothing yet, then relax further into the tapping. Relax into the night feeling, idea, or sensation like a shaking apple tree, and step beyond it to find a second feeling.

Create a word or image in that second step, and when it's clear, stop tapping. Let your hands just settle on your chest. Keep them there for the moment as we're about to tap again.

What emerges as your second idea? Tell me what it is, an image, word, or recollection. Whisper it out loud... Say it again... Sit with it without censure, measure, rule, or overrule. Open to a wider view and see what ideas enter from the sides that you don't watch. Accept and amplify that feeling, release your mind and muscles to whatever is dragged in.

Steep yourself in that place or image. A recollection of what was or might be. Place your hands back on your chest, if you have moved them to somewhere else. Although in truth, anywhere that feels resonant inside you will shake apples from the tree of thoughts.

Changing

You want to move beyond this second image to a third image or feeling, an opposite that's more or less. Tap again in alternation, one hand and then the other: TAP, tap... TAP, tap... TAP, tap...

Amplify your second thought by focus, and then attend to it's shadow. We're made of contradictions, so we always create opposites of any focus. Just sink down to relax into feeling, emotion, or association. Look for road signs and symbols, your own collage of costumes you have known.

Tell me the next word, the third word, image, vision, or idea that becomes present. Sense, or sensation, now open—time slows, gliding, almost horizontal—what's that feel like? Who is your personality that says it? What is their motive? What is their landscape? What comes next in a flash or quiet presentation? Is it full, or is it empty?

In the learning process, what comes first comes from outside. Say it to me in a whisper. Whisper it with feeling, and watch it float like a balloon above the treetops... like spilled milk across the floor... water burbling under the bridge... a horse cantering out of the barn. What ideas and images wait in the wings, on the horizon, over the rainbow, to hang under the harvest moon?

Sit with this third idea, and let your hands rest. We're done with tapping now. This little exploration of transitions, transitions that happen all the time, always transitions from one focus to the next. Relax and let your arms settle to your chest, your lap, the arms of the chair, or down beside you.

Where are you now? You've gone two associations from where you started with the night vision you began. What does this feeling now share with what you started with? Is this progress, regress, getting older or younger? Have you moved forward, sideways, parallel, or perpendicular? Might there be no difference between all of these, as they're all states of you? Is what you were, are, and are becoming really different, or is it just like the rising of a cake? A metamorphosis or a ripening? Bigger or different? Which would you prefer?

Frustration

Take this as an example. Today I wake up feeling frustrated and, lying in bed after waking, see one of my hands missing the first knuckles of two fingers. My hand is not cut or bleeding. It is intact but parts are missing. The injury was old and had healed long ago. I know I really have all my fingers, so I ask myself, "How could this happen?" I ask myself, "When did this happen?" As these thoughts and images fade, I feel my frustration between my fingers.

Before these images, it's a foreboding. Afterwards it feels pre-existing. Taking more time to drift, I refocus and settle myself. I am carrying it already, not something in the making, and I am relieved. I draw a boundary to contain it, to enforce it.

Frustrations emerge variously in my day, and I project what would have been my frustration onto my images, which are only somewhat real, and my mood remains composed. I wonder, as I might not if I didn't have an image to separate from, if this injury is perhaps quite old, more of a shadow I cast than something in the present.

Something Else

These images and textures, gossamer things—don't call them dreams—they are transitions. You have a finger on the pulse of this dream state always. You just don't have the time to dwell on these lost themes, face lifted into the present.

Let this under-dream process go on all day, at all times, in the background. The night dreams are only bigger because your censor-mind's off-duty. Associations come thicker when your mind processes them bigger, and the drill sergeant of what's now at attention has gone away.

You know reverie is sometimes inappropriate, and others won't allow you to entrance them. "Wake up!" they'll urge when you are lost, almost scared you'll take them with you. Be too obvious and they may see you as too spaced out, but too rigid and you appear heartless. You want to make some space behind your personality. Expand for yourself a bigger flexibility.

Last year, in a restaurant I was in, someone just checked out. She sat at the table, staring and unresponsive, lost somewhere no one could reach. The repeated attempts of her companion to connect broke the surface of social rhythm as a fear spread through the room, fear of a different reality, far from the mostly empty normal banter, and you could feel the disquiet settle over the room like a quiet snow.

An emergency response was called, and some others came to attend. And after a while, she came back and, escorted by her companion, walked assisted out of doors. You can imagine the relief we strangers felt!—just for a hair's breadth of attention, a moment gone too long.

And just how fragile are you, or under orders you can't recall, that you're forbidden to call timeout when the muse knocks at your door?

Come Back to Normal

Inhale to gather your deeper feelings as you left them just before. Here is the deepest idea you found, two sets of tapping from the first. Three ideas connected, perhaps appearing unrelated. Take a breath and relax into that space that makes your background. Exhale those ideas back into your muscles and your joints.

Inhale back to the second idea, the level to which your first tapping brought you, if you can remember where that was. It was the idea in between where you started and where you first peeked out above the top. Take a breath from that space. Inhale… Honor the idea as a transition, even if it's only held by travelers. Exhale… A platform on which only vagrants sleep.

And last, inhale yourself back to normal: present, whole, and clear-headed. Back to cordial conversation and thoughts that don't lead too far, so you always have the space you need for attention to the details. Engage the alert response.

There is only so much you can do awake. We think it's where our life is, but it's only a time we use for filling, coloring in last night's emotions, and collecting the new beach shells of the day.

Back now, energy in hands and feet, attention to outward motions, organized and pleasant, breathing as normal. Complete, ready, ears attuned, and eyes open.

The Path to Sleep

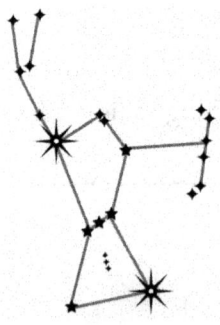

11 Dream Crafting 2: Inside of Dreams

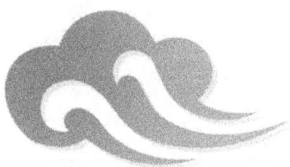

PLAYING A ROLE IN DREAMS.

Therapeutic Dreaming

The first part of the "dream crafting" topic addressed preparing dreams and preparing yourself for dreams. This part invokes the subconscious in daydreams and evokes awareness in night dreams.

There are cultures that have and still do ascribe great importance to dreams. And—though seen as superstitious—ours does, too. Whether or not we admit their importance, dreams affect us deeply.

The early Greeks practiced a healing regime called Asclepian Dream Therapy. Asclepius was the Greek demi-god of medicine and a Jesus-like healer of souls. Therapy consisted of ritual purification and an extended time in the holy chambers wrapped in furs, experiencing dreams and visions. Priests would then consider these indications before prescribing a healing regimen.

Many indigenous peoples consider dreams healing, prophetic, communications from a higher source. It's sometimes said native cultures don't dream, they have visions. From her apprenticeship in Mayan dreaming, learning traditional recall, sharing, and symbol interpretations, Barbara Tedlock calls dreams "complex psychodynamic communicative events" that create the Mayan social reality.

The Senoi tribes in the mountains of Malaysia sleep all together in family groups. They recognize shared dreaming, which means they interpret interrelated dreams as being a connected, single event experienced by two or

The Path to Sleep

more people. The Senoi use dreaming as a tool for maintaining family and social structure.

Tibetan culture includes a pre-Buddhist tradition of dream yoga, through the practice of which we can:

> "... *cultivate greater awareness during every moment of life. If we do, freedom and flexibility continually increase and we are less governed by habitual preoccupations and distractions. We develop a stable and vivid presence that allows us to more skillfully choose positive responses to whatever arises, responses that best benefit others and our own spiritual journey.*
>
> *"Eventually we develop a continuity of awareness that allows us to maintain full awareness during dream as well as in waking life. Then we are able to respond to dream phenomena in creative and positive ways and can accomplish various practices in the dream state. When we fully develop this capacity, we will find that we are living both waking and dreaming life with greater ease, comfort, clarity, and appreciation... [and we can] attain liberation from the dreaminess of ordinary life and use sleep to wake from ignorance."*

—Tenzin Wangyal Rinpoche, in *The Tibetan Yogas Of Dream And Sleep*

People of these cultures have an important place for dreams in their everyday lives. They recognize a different boundary between the dream and waking worlds. Considering these alternatives makes it clear that our boundaries are attitudes, not facts. Our view of dreams is neither scientific, certain, nor immutable.

Science and Magic

My understanding of dreams comes from the physics of how things are represented. Physics gives us ways to consider separate things that interact and are simultaneously parts of a whole. It provides models to describe unusual structures, things and events that are related but may not occur in sequence, events that affect each other strongly though are widely and unpredictably separated over time and space.

In our common use of language, events that are related but take place simultaneously at a distance from each other are not easily understood. For them we invent theories of cause and effect. Related events that lack a causal connection, or do not happen in sequence, are poorly expressed and poorly analyzed, if they're analyzed at all.

We see what we look for and consider to be real what we agree to have seen. Through this modern consensus version of reality we have created an incorrect boundary between the mental and physical worlds. The distinction between the objective physical world and the subjective mental one is a legacy rooted in the early struggle between science and religion. It is no longer helpful.

To understand dreams, we need tools to combine alternatives into a whole, especially alternatives that appear to conflict. These tools are beautifully presented to us in the mathematics of quantum systems and include wave-particle duality, self-similarity, complementarity, the breaking of symmetry, and the simultaneous expression of conflicting alternatives. These ideas pertain to all things and all systems. They are not limited to inanimate laboratory experiments.

In this material, I implicitly use ideas of transition through chaos and the structure of quantum systems. I'm not talking about what has become "quantum flapdoodle"—the misappropriation of physics to substantiate the inexplicable and erroneous—but analogies based on a deep understanding of soma and psyche. I make no effort to explain these ideas here. I simply apply them.

It will be decades, and several more generations, before these ideas are accurately understood in common use. An appreciation of these concepts has barely started to percolate into psychology, engineering, medicine, and social consciousness.

I also incorporate notions of self-healing from "energy medicine," a range of experiential mind-body approaches to healing and personal change. Energy healing is often untested, unscientific, and metaphysical, even magical. Elements of it exist in Reiki, shamanic healing, body work, medical intuition, and other approaches that use similar elements in different forms.

Ironically, there is no integrated understanding of integrative healing. These fields will eventually coalesce into a whole, like drops of oil on the surface of the water. For my purposes, I collect ideas from energy medicine like flowers, putting together those that look good.

Where science provides definition and discipline, energy medicine allows for free and undefined ideas. This freedom is a large part of all healing as personal change is largely subjective and undefined. Much of what we do here is suggestive, metaphoric, and contrived for effect. It is difficult for us to fit this within the scientific method.

Understand dreams outside of reality as you know it. Other cultural and intellectual perspectives provide alternative signposts to commonly held beliefs, some newer and some much older.

When We Dream

I object to the notion of dreaming as a separate state. I reject the idea that those states of mind in which we are physiologically asleep are our only dream states. If dreams are a resource, then why limit ourselves to when we are asleep and our dreams are the most difficult to reach? We dream all the time, asleep or awake. Let's explore and enhance this. Let's become adept at participating in the dreams we have while we're awake.

When we talk about recalling sleep dreams, we're referring to the difference between recalling nothing versus something from the time we're asleep. Throughout the day, you have daydreams, reveries, and fantasies, most of which you are only peripherally aware of and usually forget. In fact, most of these we're barely aware of at the time we're having them! Before making a big deal about our nighttime dreams, we should take our daytime dreams more seriously.

Remembering one nighttime dream is a good accomplishment, and remembering more than one from a single night is unusual. What we recall of these nighttime dreams may not be much more than a daytime reverie. It is my experience that by improving my skill at slipping in and out of daydreams, I become better at slipping in and out of night dreams. This only makes sense: If you improve your waking connection with your subconscious, then you'll retain this improved connection no matter what state you're in.

Remembering Daydreams

We typically commandeer our daydreams, not our night dreams. We're involved in long night dreams but not long daydreams. Of the two doors to greater involvement, becoming less lucid in daydreams is easier than becoming more lucid in night dreams.

To enhance your daydreams, give them time, and give them power. Set aside time to daydream, to allow yourself to daydream fully, freely, and without the interference of your conscious mind. When I give my mind this opportunity, the ideas that float through my imagination are much like those of a night's dreaming. When I intentionally hold myself in a state of reverie, stories start to form like strands of sugar on a stick in a cotton-candy machine.

Most people would rather undergo a mild electric shock than meditate for five minutes. Given this level of self-alienation, is it any surprise that the sleeping dreamtime our bodies force upon us leave strange, confusing, and quickly forgotten memories?

Improve your ability to daydream. I'm not talking about becoming absent by taking more naps, and I'm not talking about controlling your mind through meditation, though both of these may be steps toward deeper daydreaming, a greater non-awareness.

I'm talking about placing yourself in a trance during the comfortable part of the day. Allow yourself to remain undisturbed for at least ten minutes. Ask your conscious mind to remain quiet, in the background but not silent, just listening and watching as ideas float and build like clouds in your mind. Have you ever done this? This is the objective of "Daydreaming," the first exercise in this chapter.

Remembering Night Dreams

Whatever purpose dreams serve, remembering them seems unnecessary. This begs the question of whether remembering dreams is even a good idea or just a disturbance. Is there anything wrong with the way we have patterned our lives, a pattern and a schedule that causes us to forget our dreams?

Perhaps we should be waking up gradually, and in that way have better dream recall. Does our sleeping and waking routine, dictated by what is socially accepted and economically required, create underlying problems? I think it does because improving dream recall also improves sleep. That is, weak dream recall correlates with generally poor sleep, and poor sleep is partly due to the way we pattern our lives.

Dreams are not designed to be remembered consistently and in detail. They are designed to have a variable effect. This is my opinion. There is a healthy interaction between our conscious and our subconscious minds, and poor sleep and poor dream recall reflects an unhealthy loss of contact.

Recalling dreams does not disrupt the purpose of dreaming. Occasionally we remember detailed dreams. This is more likely when we have woken ourselves up in order to do so. In most cases, we recall little of our dreams, if we remember them at all.

Certainly, one can train oneself for better dream recall, but might this border on interference? And if one trains in this way, then recall grades into intentional lucid and controlled dreaming. Taken to the extreme, this certainly is disruptive to the normal dream pattern and the mostly subconscious world of dreams.

I sound as if I'm against recalling one's dreams, but this is not true. I am against arguments that entreat your subconscious to establish rational lines of communication with you. This borders on interrogation.

What I support is a dialog between your conscious and subconscious. If that dialog results in greater dream recall, then it's right and natural. And if that dialog results in something else, then that result is right and natural. How will you know which is right for you? You develop a dialog, and then you'll see. With that goal in mind, the goal of giving you the tools to better communicate with your subconscious, we pursue the techniques of lucid dreaming.

An unattributed post at The Lucidity Institute (http://www.lucidity.com), borrowing from the work of Stephen LaBerge, comments:

> To increase your dream recall is to remind yourself as you are falling asleep that you wish to awaken fully from your dreams and remember them… it may help to tell yourself you will have interesting, meaningful dreams.

View dream recall as the avoidance of forgetting as opposed to an act of remembering. In an anonymous 1989 piece called "How to remember your dreams," published by The Lucidity Institute in *Nightlight* (1) 1, we're told:

> A major cause of dream forgetting is interference from other thoughts competing for your attention. Therefore, let your first thought upon awakening be, 'What was I just dreaming?' Before attempting to write down the dream, go over the dream in your mind, re-telling the dream

story to yourself.

DO NOT MOVE from the position in which you awaken, and do not think of the day's concerns. Cling to any clues of what you might have been experiencing—moods, feelings, fragments of images, and try to rebuild a story from them. When you recall a scene, try to recall what happened before that, and before that, reliving the dream in reverse. If after a few minutes, all you remember is a mood, describe it in a journal.

Finally, we're told to consider what dreams we may have had, even if we're unsure if we actually had them:

If you can recall nothing, try imagining a dream you might have had—note your present feelings, list your current concerns to yourself, and ask yourself, 'Did I dream about that?' Even if you can't recall anything in bed, events or scenes of the day may remind you of something you dreamed the night before... record whatever you remember.

This raises an intriguing point. If a dream is a thought like any other, then how much of it is imagined and how much is remembered? Memory and imagination are always intermixed. The recollection of imagination is much the same as the imagination of a recollection. Is there any real difference between falsely remembering a dream you didn't have and truly remembering one you did?

The real question may not be whether you can remember your dreams but whether you can regain that creative state. That is your goal. The "reality" of your dream and its recall may not matter. The upwelling of ideas from your subconscious is your dialog. It may be just as well to have that dialog in the moment as to remember it from a dream before.

Dreams are not a realm of unconstrained creativity and impulsiveness. Creativity and restraint remain under your control even when you feel lost or frightened. We don't have a way to measure one person's creativity against another's, but you can measure it for yourself. You can ask yourself how creatively you're willing to think.

You cannot expect any vision of what you are not yet able to see, but you can get answers in the form of inclinations, intuitions, sensations, and expectations. You must understand that in realms where you cannot yet think in words—whether they be your dream or waking state—inclination, intuition, sensation, and expectation are mechanisms of thought and the currency of the answers you receive.

The goal of dream awareness is to change your future. You do this by finding new feelings, thoughts, and memories, or a new space of self that welcomes novelty. You do not force yourself into a different state. You create for yourself a different process, a process in which you accept a therapeutic role in calling in those forces that are in you, or operate through you, to address issues that are beyond you.

To converse with your subconscious is to accept the role of being your own doctor, in which case the old adage, "The doctor who treats herself has a fool for a patient," could not be more true. It is a dissociated role, as you must be both or several—certainly the doctor and the fool, but also the angels, demons, ancestors, and others, too.

Creating Dreams

The goal in therapeutic dreaming is to call upon inner forces to provide a different, richer, and more powerful perspective to life's issues. You evoke these forces by stirring issues from within your body, deeply feeling and visualizing in your mind as you go to sleep. Create a state of mind that is in touch with the issues that move you strongly.

Shaping the content of your dreams begins with a focus of intention and expectation well before you go to sleep. Your expectation of your dreams plays a role in your waking life as you register certain feelings and events for "sleeping on" in the near future. Recognize issues you want to explore further in dreams. Let sleep and dreaming be a repository for concerns and emotions that build during the day. Issues that might otherwise be lost for lack of contemplation are tagged for review in sleep.

Start the process by setting your intention to dream about these issues. Create an intention deep enough to generate feelings even without your awareness. What about this issue or need draws you forward? Is it who you want to be, or feel, or think?

Close your eyes to look over your emotional landscape, your dream landscape, and cast the seeds of this becoming. Feel right with their settling.

Dream Crafting 2: Inside of Dreams

This must feel right or the intention will not take root.

Rehearse your dreams as daydreams while still awake. Build high expectations and a greater sense of importance. Build an integrated view of what's possible or what's missing. You don't know when, how, or if... and you don't need to. You're not out to find answers; you're out to ask questions, to put these before your higher self. Forming vibrant questions is the point. You put these out, and someone else puts the answers together or simply throws the questions away.

See yourself moving forward toward two paths: one up and the other down, beginning together and leading apart. The path up is constructive, a path of recovery and recreating, reforming and resetting. The path down is destructive, a path of dis-creation and discovery, deforming and disassembling. Both can be positive or negative. Each can be both. Judgement doesn't play a role. Be open.

These are paths of connection you can change by intention and force of will. Work with the energies you can change, and change what's within your reach. Dwell on the negative until it softens like butter, mixed with the lard of the positive, and cut in the flour of potential until all is coarse and granular. Add milk and honey. The dream does the baking.

Write an engaging story, a mystery you can't put down. Create your own anticipation for a process with a motion of its own, a movement toward change, enhancing and revising. Confront and conquer danger, even if you feel too small for the task. Do not be a victim. Advance toward love and respect. Positive energy radiates from your hands and eyes, emerging as light, heat, or liquid. Create space for a positive outcome.

The negative manifests as strife, fear, illness, or disease. Diminish the negative by dissolution, disassembly, detachment, disposal, change, reconstruction, deconstruction, cleansing, clearing, reviving, decaying, allowing, admitting, inviting, assisting, vitalizing, gratifying, forgiving, explaining, releasing, excusing, or simply paying off. Give these elements their due. Enable them to leave.

Let's imagine your actions are to heal yourself now, in this relaxed state. Let this become a memory that you can access in your dreamtime. Let this become a guide or template for where to find your healing energy and how to focus and direct it.

Lucid Dreams

The goal of therapeutic dreaming is insight. The goal of lucid therapeutic dreaming is to ask for insight while you're dreaming. You will not know the situation or the question until you are in the dream, so you need to aim to have enough awareness to ask the right question at the time.

There are several confusions about lucid dreaming. The first is that anyone can learn to lucid dream. While hypnotic training has the highest success rate in teaching lucid dreaming, half of those who engage in multi-week programs still report no lucid dreams. The evidence is that half of those who try do not learn to lucid dream.

The second confusion is the idea that creating a dream, imagining you're lucid while dreaming, and actually being lucid in a dream are different things. They are not. They are all aspects of the same process. It's important that you do not judge your success in these tasks separately. Think of lucid dreaming as a process, not an outcome. Engage the process and accept the result.

The third confusion is that we understand lucidity. We assume we are lucid when awake, but we are not. Normal waking state awareness is narrowly focused, limited, and transient. We believe we share our common awakeness with others, but it is not even that. Develop the habit of questioning the reality of your waking state and you will become more self-aware in your dreaming state.

Lucid dreamers are not fully aware even when they believe themselves to be. This suggests that you are not really, fully aware even when you are awake. People with a variety of awarenesses, personalities, and degrees of mental health march in the parade of our consensus reality, but beyond basic physics, we do not share the same world. There is not one world to be lucid of.

How to Lucid Dream

Paul Tholey's technique, presented in the 1980s, includes the following guidelines of what to do while awake:

1. **Are you dreaming now?** Ask yourself whether or not you are dreaming at numerous times during the day. Ask it whenever something surprising or improbable occurs, or whenever you experience powerful emotions.

2. **Imagine you're dreaming**. Imagine you're in a dream state and everything you perceive, including your own body, is merely a dream.
3. **Recognize dream events**. If you have dream experiences that never occur in a waking state, such as floating or flying, then while you're awake, intensely imagine having these experiences while telling yourself that you're dreaming.
4. **Expect lucidity**. Go to sleep thinking you're going to attain awareness while dreaming. Avoid being analytical while thinking this thought and instead let it reside as a feeling. This is especially effective when you have just awakened in the early morning and feel you're about to fall asleep again.
5. **Have a signal**. Resolve to carry out a particular action while dreaming. Simple motions are sufficient.

The following indications apply to your actions within a dream. These are a westernization of practices ascribed to the Malaysian Senoi.

- **Conquer danger**. Assert yourself. Do not become a victim of any situation.
- **Accept pleasure**. Reject the notion of pleasure as self-indulgent or indecent because pleasure is therapeutic; it helps you love and respect yourself. Without this, you cannot love or respect others.
- **Achieve a positive outcome**. Dream reality reacts directly to the quality of your thoughts. Dreams are a training ground to see the results of your thinking. Fearful thoughts produce nightmares. Loving thoughts build empathy and affection in your personality. A solution-oriented approach changes your dream landscape accordingly.

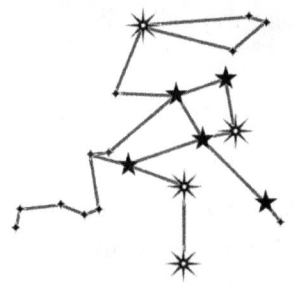

The Path to Sleep

Hypnotic Session 21

Daydreaming

Audio file at: https://www.mindstrengthbalance.com/path-to-sleep-audio/

This is an easy exercise if you relax completely. Remember how you start a daydream? Something breaks your attention and triggers a new line of thought. Relax your body, your nerves, and your mind. The hardest part of daydreaming is holding the images so that the thin rivers merge to form a narrative.

Remember when you were bored? Maybe it was in a classroom when you were a kid, or a conference room, or doing repetitive work. Make that feeling now. You are in a classroom where you don't want to be, bored by what has no meaning. You are in a conference of reviews that have no point or direction. You are shuffling and filing, doing taxes, tabulating numbers, and organizing receipts. Let me bore you to distraction.

One hundred notices, confirmations, informationals, and orientations.

Ninety-nine reminders, fliers, receipts, advertisements, claims.

Ninety-eight sheets of numbers, tallies, testimonies, postponements.

Ninety-seven envelops, addresses, redirects, and referrals.

Ninety-six items for entry, business cards, transcriptions, corrections.

Ninety-five customer lists, inventories, product codes, serial numbers.

Ninety-four phone numbers, emails, websites, important contacts.

Ninety-three essential items, important issues, things not to forget.

Ninety-two grocery lists, shopping lists, lists of words, parts, and assemblies.

Ninety-one things to do, things you'll never remember.

Ninety people you'd like to connect with...

Who is someone you'd really like to connect with? Is this a person you know, have known, would like to know, would like to know better, or would like to meet? Hold them in your mind's eye. Are they looking at you or at something else? Draw their attention to you, as it once was, could have been, or may yet be. Feel the connection: a spark, catching to turn over, to ignite or recognize. Consider it.

Daydreams start like confetti, thoughts of one word each. Hold them in your mind until they become a turbulence of butterflies and moths, ideas and images made from tatters and tippets. With deep and quiet relaxation, these ribbons weave into a story.

Daydreams have the mysterious quality of falling apart if you look at them while they're forming. You must keep them in the corner of your eye, without attachment or involvement, without thinking about them.

Daydreams form like snowflakes in a cloud, growing around a seed as a memory, an idea, image, or feeling. They grow quickly, almost too quickly. You must slow them down, slow them down.

Imagine you're in a wide grass field on the first day of winter. The sky is a thick white, and there is a cloud all around you and above you. You can barely see the edge of the field as surrounding treetops are lost in white. The sound is muffled and still. The air is crisp on your skin, dry and prickling. And there is a blanket of silence that you can almost hear coming, coming from above you, the sense of sound being sucked away as the first snowflakes of winter begin to swirl about you.

Think about the last twenty-four hours, your last full-day cycle. Think about how it started. Maybe it was today or maybe yesterday.

Who did you see? Recall the scene. Maybe it's a face, an empty room, or a room with a person you can't see. What did it feel like? Hold on to a picture with a feeling.

What happened then? Move on to later. Something happened next. Maybe not immediately, but later. What comes to mind?

It's odd how insignificant pictures present themselves: entering a parking lot, drinking from a cup, looking out a window, passing through a doorway, the feeling you get when your phone rings, a dog crossing the road, a flock of birds.

What happened last evening? The sun was setting, the day already over. How did that feel? What emotions textured past, almost gone before you noticed, like a change in the surface of the road.

These are the snowflakes, all around you.. See yourself from the viewpoint of the snowflakes, circling in helical patterns as if down a spiral slide, a slide at a playground, a slide at a water park, falling, swinging as if on a string, and there is you down below looking up. And with each rotation, spinning down, you rotate into view and then out again. And what do you look like? What are you wearing?

And each snowflake is a thought, one of your thoughts, one of your memories from the day gone past. Each snowflake, an idea or image repeating: parking lot, window, doorway, phone call, dog bark. And these snowflakes circle down, drawn toward you by your focus and attention, now in a whispering blizzard of a whispered silence, circling your head like moths, circling around you. A warm candle in a cold winter field. Circling around you.

And as they circle, entraining behind them is a trail of other snowflakes, each growing into ideas and feelings, hanging snowflakes of yesterday's images. Pick one that keeps calling you. Imagine a moth, not one of the little moths that live indoors, but a great wild furry moth that could have been a fairy in another life: Atlas, Comet, Emperor, Luna. Colorful, huge antennaed, with a single mind and kaleidoscope eyes.

This moth carries a story written on its wings, on the scales of its wings. This story starts with a single word, thought, or picture and repeats in greater detail on each of its scales, its hundreds of scales, reflecting and refracting. Its hundreds of thousands of scales so delicate, so easily brushed off with a touch, which is why you should not touch it, but watch it turn and shape into ideas and feelings.

What idea has found you, to circle about your head? This from which your dreams are made, rising like a cake in the oven of your sleep. Rising now.

Dream Crafting 2: Inside of Dreams

Take off and stow your judging mind. Set it by the door, and let ideas pile up like snowflakes on a windless early snowstorm afternoon. They won't last. The sun will soon return, and the now white trees will be gray again in minutes. You only have a moment to collect them.

Take this idea, and let me count from five to one, keeping your ears busy and the hound of your attention occupied.

Five. The idea that came to you with details that have meaning.

Four. An idea that whispered recollections and meaning.

Three. Reminders, recollections, and emotions that trail behind it.

Two. From its images and pictures that grow like shoots to unlikely places.

One. A sidewalk sketch, magic, and imagination. Things, places, people, and pictures.

Let this vision, feeling, sit comfortably, like swings set in motion, resonating as long as you don't touch it. Swing, roll, drift, rock, and slide into a sense of mindlessness, watching whatever comes up, out, and past you. Quietly watch without judgment the sensical conclusions mixed with nonsense rolling past a landscape in your mind, your calm, relaxed state of mind, clear or crazy headed. No judgement's needed when no understanding is presumed. Swing, drift, roll, rock, slide, drill, and tumble. Easy, nice, good, calm, and patient.

Let me ask your higher guidance. Let me call it in by name. What is the name you give your higher guidance? There is none, I would expect, but I call it just the same, and I ask it, "What is this image? How will this whisper collect and vote itself into existence? Why will it, when will it, and what does it mean?"

Five. How will these whispers of recollections rearrange themselves?

Four. Where does the idea come from to join them together, to make a stew of ideas?

Three. Will they find themselves in your dreams, now, later, or ever?

Two. From images and pictures growing like shoots and surprises.

One. Like a picture book, a painting, or a poem.

You lose yourself in these thoughts, as you want to. Release the eye of your control. Just as you often try to find an understanding, there is no reason to do this now. Let ideas float in fractured form, well-packed or even broken, no instructions or insurance, no expectation, no hurry, no need. Relaxed and attentive.

You lose yourself in the thoughts tracing through the back of your mind. Some coursing jet trails over the puffy clouds of feelings and emotions. Others tumbling softly, building up or evaporating down, shifting, coming and going like bubbles, like snatches of music, like sensations.

If we've kindled a fire or primed a pump, then let the fire burn and the pump spill ideas that flow through your head like water and fire, some cool and others hotter, some closer and others far away.

Listen to my patter just to have something to push against. It doesn't mean anything; it just holds a place to keep our mind's eye calm, scratching behind the ears of our mind's eye, rubbing the dog's belly of our perseverating mind whose thinking is mostly reflex, like the tremor in the dog's leg, lying on its back, scratching at the air.

Relax and give yourself a moment of blank thought, bright as daylight, gray and cloudy twilight, or the rich dark of insight.

Return to the normal time, the time we consent is awareness, the you that we agree is who you appear to be. Put that back on with little need for thinking, and so you come back. Return to yourself with your daydream mind intact, ready, operating always, a you who's better now to hear it. Always.

I'll count from one to five, counting from deep relaxation back to the present and its commonplace preparation, consideration, and deliberation. And when I get to three, you'll be feeling your hands and your feet. And when I get to four, but I have not gotten there yet, you'll feel the live energy in your lungs, throat, face, and eyes. And when I reach five, you'll be feeling refreshed and relaxed, more balanced, and more comfortable than before.

One. Recalling your mind and presentation, yourself, personality, and surroundings.

Two. Letting my voice drift into the background and your voice resume its echo.

Three. Feeling your body, all around your body, your hands and feet, chest, sides, arms, head, and shoulders.

Four. Focusing on your own energy, the rhythm of your pulse, the swelling of your breath, the tingling of your skin.

And Five. Feeling refreshed and relaxed, balanced and comfortable, vibrating. Back, present, eyes open, awake and aware.

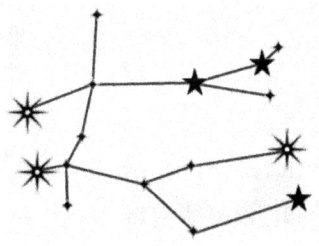

Hypnotic Session 22

Therapeutic Lucid Dreaming

Audio file at: https://www.mindstrengthbalance.com/path-to-sleep-audio/

Look straight ahead of you. Then, without moving your head, what do you see in front of you? What if you move your eyes to either side? What is beyond the walls around you? What would you see if you were one hundred feet in the air looking out toward the horizon?

Relax and take a deep breath. Inhale... Exhale... And remember when you were in the water, or on the water, floating in the ocean, a lake, on a raft, or a boat. And if you can't remember exactly, then imagine a warm bath heating and relaxing your joints and muscles. Lifting you beyond gravity, beyond weight, and beyond concern.

Feel the water lifting your shoulders, taking the weight off your back. Feel your feet weightless.

Feel your hands surrounded by light and warmth, encased in auras, like clouds of ball lightning, full of energy.

Hear what's around you: my voice, the ticking of a clock, the humming of a motor, the movement of air, the quiet in the room.

Imagine I'm slicing a fresh lemon, and you can smell it. Can you recall the smell of freshly cut lemon? What does your tongue have to say about it?

I have a bouquet of fresh red roses. I unwrap them, and their odor wafts through the room. Can you recall the sweet fruit smell of roses? Imagine the smell of pine, the balsam fir at Christmas shopping for a tree, and the smell as you run your fingers across the needles? The smell of pine sap, or oranges, or rain.

Relax your neck, your jaw, your back and spine. Inhale... And exhale all the tension in these bones and muscles. Imagine we are driving a car on a dark night, and I am with you. You're tired, and you pull over. I get behind the wheel so you can take a short rest. You are lucid now but not dreaming.

Imagine you are dreaming of sitting in your car. I have taken over driving, and we are back on the road. You are resting, feeling the vibration of the car and the road, the dull hum of the engine and the roar of the road. Imagine your are lucid in a dream that you are imagining.

I will offer you ideas to keep in the back of your mind. These ideas help your transition from being passive in a dream to becoming aware that you are dreaming and asserting your own identity, even there. The ideas are about becoming lucid.

I will give you suggestions of how you will resolve to think and act in a dream. The suggestions are true whether you are lucid or not. Part of your dream is written before it starts while you are awake. Part of it is written before it starts while you are asleep. And part of it is written after it starts while you are dreaming. Whether you are lucid or not may or may not determine how your dreams end.

Recognize right thinking and acting in dreams—thinking straight and clear—as in life, as something you do regardless of who you are, where you are, or when, whether you are lucid or not, awake or asleep, dead or alive. Adopt right thought and action everywhere, and it will be in your dreams, as well.

Here are the ideas you are to follow simply throughout the day: simple thoughts that are just for you to remember, ideas that you recollect whenever you switch gears or take a breath, and ideas that can float through your mind, both serious and humorous, dull, vague, focused, or refined.

Are you dreaming now? Are you perceiving what's in your mind, or are you imagining it? What does this mean? Get in this habit. When something strikes you—something strong, an emotion or a feeling—ask, "Is this is a perception or my imagination?"

Get in the habit of asking if this is real. How do you really feel? And are you indulging in a dream, or are you really in possession of yourself? Who is in possession of you now? Is it the familiar you or an unfamiliar you?

The Path to Sleep

Whenever something odd or out of the ordinary occurs, ask this: ask if you are dreaming.

Relax more deeply now. Take a breath. Inhale… Exhale… Sink more deeply, spinning like a leaf or a maple seed twirling on its rotor blade, spinning from the treetops in a sunshine cloud of skies.

Imagine you're dreaming. Imagine this now, looking through the trees to a blue sky with high white wisps. Imagine other daytime scenes that happen all the time: walking out your door, getting in your car, standing on the street, buying groceries, watching traffic in your rear-view mirror. And in these times and places, imagine they are dreams. How would they be different?

You give them a momentary glance, and then back to your inner thoughts. You check the mirror, your footstep, or the position of the sun, and then you go back to your thoughts and reveries. Imagine this a dream, and consider how similar this is to waking life.

Sense your body, the shape of your head, the width of your shoulders, the size of your ribs, the shape of your breast, the curve of your spine. If this were a dream, would it not seem just the same? It might. It might not. If this were a dream, what would you feel next? Attend to the next sensation. Sense your feet, or look at your hands. Imagine these, and recognize them in your imagination. Is it a dream, or are you awake? Are they different? Can you wake up in either of them?

Move your right forefinger. Squint your eyes. Pout your lips. Take a breath. Inhale… Exhale… Let your mind go blank for a moment. Relax and sink into the chair. Relax and sink. Feel the texture under your fingertips.

What strange things have you done in your dreams? Have you flown? Sometimes I do, and other times I almost do. I float. I often jump down whole flights of stairs to land perfectly, easily, twenty or forty feet down at the bottom. I do this often. I do this when I'm awake, or I think I do. Am I? Are you? What do you do in your dreams that is such a relief?

Do that now in your imagination. If you fly, then fly. If you see far away or around corners, then do that. If you teleport, then do that. Pass through walls. Hear other people think. Heal yourself miraculously. Do that.

These are dream things. You are dreaming when you do this. Awake or asleep, these are dream abilities. See yourself doing your dream ability, your sleep ability, and tell yourself you will know this when it happens in a dream.

And when you know you are dreaming, then you know you are simply imagining, and you can set the topic of conversation. You can ask the dream to speak to you, as if it were an artist's canvas that hears and responds, because that is what it is, and you can talk in it, with it, to it, and it will answer you as the voice, the face, and the hands of your imagination.

When these ordinary and amazing things happen, you are dreaming. Practice now. It's not so easy to be aware and in control and also imagining and watching. Becoming lucid in dreams isn't much easier than becoming lucid and watching your awake state thoughts form, but it isn't harder either.

Try it now. Imagine you're on a small boat pushing off into a lake. You're with a companion and a picnic basket. And now your boat, passenger, and basket are floating in the water, in the lake. And now your boat, passenger, and basket are floating in the air above the lake.

And now you stand in the boat, and you say, "A beautiful island," and an island appears, and all of a sudden, you are sitting on the ground watching a sunset form over the lake.

Wave your hand and the island becomes a forest. The forest forms a road, and you wish a car to appear and it does. You get in, and you drive off into the sunset. It's hard to both imagine and control. It takes effort, but you can do it.

Relax. Take a break. Let your legs settle. Make yourself comfortable. Where are you tense? Your neck, your back, your jaw, your shoulders? Relax those. Let them down. Let them out. Balance your neck. Release the tension in your neck. Release more deeply, and let your breath out. Let your mind out.

You can expect to be lucid. Imagine a dream, a ridiculous dream. You're in a place, and it's not familiar. You're with people, but you cannot see them. You're traveling, but you don't know where. You see yourself, but you don't know how you got here, or why, or where you're going.

And when you do, it's no big deal. It's just a moment of novelty, an idea from another place, a movement out of normal, and a situation with a message. You will know it's a dream. You know it's a dream. You will have known it's a dream. It's obviously a dream, and you're comfortable in it.

You can tell the others, but they likely will not listen. It's not their world, just yours. You'll look for those who do know. Those are the ones to talk to. They know what goes on behind the scenes, beyond the script, outside the set. They know the higher worlds or else they might direct you there. That's where you'll go, to the higher worlds, to look out over the hills of possibility, the mountains of certitude, and the ocean of wisdom.

Have a signal for when you get there, to recognize you're dreaming, knowing you can look for another path. Signal to yourself simply. Be quiet and reserved. Just look at your hands or feet, see yourself in a mirror, scratch your nose, lift a finger, make a fist, squint your eyes, look left and right. You might say out loud, "I am dreaming," or "I can change things," or "It doesn't have to be this way."

Don't interrupt your dream; work with it. Don't be a bother or a nuisance. Part of being lucid is being sensitive. It may be that your being lucid is allowed because it serves the dream's purpose. And the dream has a purpose, and it's not yours to hijack.

Be positive, speak quietly, and be present and attentive. Overcome danger, accept pleasure, and move toward the positive. There will be things you need to hear, opportunities to speak, and actions you can take.

Being lucid is a role like any role, and you must apply for it and apply yourself to it. In what dream would you be comfortably lucid? In what dream would you be helpful? In what dream would your being lucid accomplish what you could not accomplish otherwise?

Being lucid is rare for me, and in most of my dreams, being lucid would be inappropriate. If I were lucid in most of my dreams, being the thinker that I am, I would avoid the unpleasant and resolve the unresolvable. That may not be right. Do I need to experience the unpleasant? Do I need to accept the unresolvable? Being lucid is to have a narrow and willful view, and dreams are often just the opposite: wide and will-less. That's how you move to new territory, experience new sensations, and feel new emotions.

You will be lucid in a dream that is safe and comfortable. You will be lucid in a dream where you can be a "student driver," and you won't hit anything. You will be lucid, and it will be safe, and comfortable, and positive. And if you don't find yourself lucid, then know there is a reason for it, that it would not be right, or safe, or helpful.

Offer your services as a lucid dreamer, and accept what comes. Release your lucidity now, and let your intentions relax. Let yourself drift away from your sense of self and purpose, and float in that amniotic sea in-between there and here, real and imagined, the open space, the field, the ocean.

Bob up to the surface of the ocean, and breathe air again. You're a walking animal, feet on the ground. Feel the weight of your feet and energy rising up from your feet.

Your hands touch. Sense through touch what your new hands feel. Warm or cool, what's beneath your fingers? What's around your hands?

Ears hear. What do you hear around you? My voice, the static in your ears, air moving, the creak of movement. Can you hear your own pulse? Can you hear what's far beyond: birds singing, trees moving, the atmosphere, the sun?

Tongue tastes, nose smells. What can you taste and smell now? Take a deep breath. Inhale... Exhale... What can you smell? Is it new air or air that you're used to? Can you remember any smells, any good smells, like pine or roses, oranges or rain?

The Path to Sleep

And open your eyes and look. Without moving your head, what do you see in front of you? And what if you move your eyes to either side? What is beyond the walls around you? What would you see if you were one hundred feet in the air?

Bring these all together: sight, sound, taste, and touch. Take a breath and be present, awake and alert, contained, comfortable, safe, and positive, as you want to be always, awake or asleep, in daydreams, in night dreams, and in no dreams.

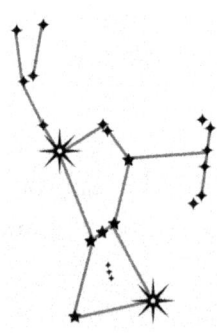

12 Wakefulness

BEING AWAKE AND BECOMING ALERT.

Wakefulness

Awake is a state of being aware and responsive, but it only requires minimal degrees of either. You're awake whether you're stepping out of bed or stepping off the high diving board, though your sense of being present differs. Being awake sets a low standard.

It depends on what you aim to do or where you're going with it. If you're tossing around in bed late at night, neither asleep nor awake, or waiting for motivation to get started, then getting out of that "excluded middle" is what you want. "Waking up" means activating your thinking mind, something you struggle to do in those halfway states.

Being alert is relative. You're alert relative to what's going on around you, being attentive or paying attention both to what is happening, and what might happen. You're awake and engaged with something in particular, such as driving or listening. You have a degree of control and response. You're awake, but not alert, when distracted, entranced, or depressed. Being alert sets a higher standard than being awake.

I'm approaching these states in terms of frequencies, and the frequencies of being alert differ from the frequencies of being awake. Alertness requires waking up and clearing the brain fog, but it requires more than that.

Stages of Awareness

We can distinguish stages of sleep according to brainwaves and your subjective report upon waking up. Could we distinguish stages of wakefulness according to brainwaves and your subjective report? That's basically what we do, but we don't call these "stages" of being awake we call them states of awareness.

What if they really were stages? What if there are different levels of wakefulness that are normal, healthy, and necessary, and you progress through them, in order to reach higher levels of wakefulness? If this were the case, then we would not say that people are different and some are more "with it" than others. We might say some people wake up more fully and others inhabit a dysregulated wakefulness. We might send them to be tested in "Wake Labs," to be fitted with breathing machines, drugs, implants, or the like.

I conjecture all states of alertness build on a basic state of wakefulness. Obviously, being alert requires being awake. From teaching people to manage their brainwaves, I have observed a basic awake state. Just as there are distinct brainwaves in sleep, there are basic brainwave patterns for being awake.

I take this point of view, not because it's proved, but because we can talk about frequencies of wakefulness, free from the discussion of "higher consciousness." We're talking about wakefulness, and wakefulness exists on a spectrum of sensitivity and engagement. We can train ourselves to be more awake and more alert, and there is nothing moral or saintly about it.

You began this project focusing on sleep, and it's fair to assume that's your interest. But I suggest you cannot understand, perfect, or manage your sleep patterns without also accepting responsibility for your patterns of wakefulness. We've got two issues here: The first is better management of our awake state so that we can sleep better. The second is better management of our asleep state so that we can be more awake.

I feel we have already addressed the first of these. We've explored patterns, habits, intentions, and expectations in order to improve our sleep. Here I want to explore the spectrum in the other direction, toward greater alertness.

Let's consider two parts, or aspects, of wakefulness. The first is being awake and maintaining wakefulness. The second is being alert and maintaining alertness. For both cases we focus on frequency and intention.

Frequency and Intention

Just being awake doesn't amount to much. It's like being in neutral rather than drive. Your motor is running, but you're not going anywhere. A person who's awake but not alert is in a daze, and, until they come out of it, they aren't responsive. Waking up is the first important step to being conscious.

There are many states of alertness, and I'm considering only one: the state of physical engagement with your environment. This is not high spirit or intellect, and it has a kind of tunnel vision. Being engaged in driving, running, and other automatic actions involves finely tuned, complex coordination, but not inspiration, creativity, memory, or analysis. These are not states of brilliant alertness.

We could take these exercises and explore higher states of alertness, and we'd move to and through higher states of awareness. I don't know if the techniques we use here would be sufficient. Perhaps somewhat. Let's first focus on building awareness into alertness. This is the topic of the first exercise called "On Becoming Alert."

It would be nice if we could dial in alertness by turning a knob. We can chemically amplify arousal, but alertness is more than one-dimensional. When we're falling asleep many things are happening, and if we're not falling asleep it's because many things are not happening. Just as we've worked on many dimensions to make sleep happen, so we have to build a foundation if we're to become more alert.

Building a naturally alert and wakeful state when you feel that you're falling asleep takes work, and it doesn't happen instantly. Build the foundational frequencies of alertness, and alertness will come online. It will crawl out of the fog, but give it a chance. Things have to fall into place.

And there's always the possibility that you really do need a rest, a nap, or a break. Be reasonable. This is all about how your body works when it works correctly. If you cannot shake the need to sleep, then don't try to shake it. If you're driving, pull over. Close your eyes. Your mind and body may need to drop into lower frequencies before rebounding into alertness.

Higher States

All our states need preparation and require patience. They are different combinations of frequencies, and each frequency needs to find its cadence in you. It is literally a resonance, like a spinning top, and it needs to find a balance

The Path to Sleep

without resistance. It's the lack of combining the necessary tempos that keeps you from these states, be they deeper sleep or higher awareness.

In the first exercise, we build a basic alert state on three frequencies. Play with these tempos yourself, and you'll experience other states of alertness. Speed them up. Slow them down. The results will move you along a scale, across states with similar structures. You'll find views that are higher and lower, wider and narrower, all within the sense of who you are and how you present yourself. These are normal states.

There are other states, too, and other frequencies, and those states also develop with time, patience, and practice. There are frequencies you may need to let go of that you cannot. Much attention is given to reaching new heights of liberation when the problem is releasing old lows of bondage. These are frequencies, too.

I'd like to explore this idea. I'd like to see if we can find and feel the underlying frequencies of our attention and release them, but we cannot leave ourselves with nothing, so we'll have to substitute something else.

In the next exercise, I make the small request that you locate some of the frequencies of who you are and let them go. We all have these frequencies. They are what make some people resonate with you while other people are dissonant. They are what make you comfortable and open with some, and impatient with or indifferent to others. They can turn you on or turn you off.

I think you know what these frequencies are. At least, you'd certainly know them if they were not there. You'd feel lost. You might feel annoyed or frightened by their absence. I'm asking you to feel alone because that's what it feels like when you let go of who you are. That's what it feels like when you cease broadcasting your signature frequencies.

Maybe you can't do this. Maybe it's too much to ask. That's your choice. Know only that this is an offer. Join me in the experiment.

To make it easier, I'll give you other frequencies, frequencies I suspect are outside your range of personality. Some very high and others very low. I'm using tones here, rather than tempos, because I can't drum fast enough or slow enough to get outside the tempos of your personality.

The object of the second exercise called "Invitation" is simple to state but hard to achieve. The object is nothing: being nothing and feeling from nowhere.

Wakefulness

I don't know what this will mean, if you'll accept it, or what it will give you, but I know that changing your awareness will require something new. If you intend to find something, and you can, then you will.

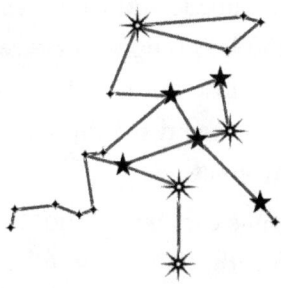

Hypnotic Session 23

On Becoming Alert

Audio file at: https://www.mindstrengthbalance.com/path-to-sleep-audio/

Drop into a relaxed state. Open the spigot of a huge bucket of warm energy above you, letting a slow and scintillating syrup warm your head, run down your back, and glue you to your chair. Glue your hands down, glue your eyes down, like it's a warm weight running down your legs and feet, on and into the earth.

You're half here and half somewhere else, somewhere nearby. Remain present and listening, watching. Let your tongue lie heavy, your jaw drop, and your throat feel warm. Let that warmth spread down your neck to bloom and blossom across your shoulders, penetrating warm oil into the hinges and ribs, down your arms to dissolve the bones in your wrists and hands. All warm now and flexible, smooth, calm, and heavy.

Unlike our other exercises aiming toward sleep, let's assume you're already somewhat sleepy, relaxed at least, and also somewhat mentally tired. Certainly you can remember or pretend that state where there was just too much happening, too much to remember, too much going on, and it seemed like you were looking for a brief time out, just a foothold, or even a brief pause to collect yourself. You can always use a pause, so take a moment now to just unburden yourself of all that's going on in and around you.

Fold yourself in like an omelette, a blintz, a crepe, an hor d'oeuvre, or a burrito, with your shell on the outside and your energy inside yourself. Draw your mental curtains, and let's reboot ourselves, starting from our resting state. Maybe that's eyes closed or eyes open, maybe it's drifting and halfway here, or maybe it's present and slightly spaced out, following the textures and landscapes of my voice.

Take a breath. Feel your lungs expand… And then exhale and let your chest contract. On the next breath, I'd like you to feel the slight pressure of your heart beating as you inhale. It's not the sense of a full cycle but rather a pulsing pressure, like someone leaning lightly on the other side of a door that you're leaning on, a kind of rocking motion. Feel that as you inhale, and notice how that sensation fades as you exhale.

Pay attention to your pulse when your inhale and feel its texture. Its texture is the tone of a muscle, like when your arms are tired, your pulse may be sharp-edged. Relax your chest, your breath, to soften your pulse. Make the load light and the rhythm smooth. Tension is a fast frequency, and you want to build awakeness on the slower frequencies: the breath, the pulse, and double times, as we explore.

Start with your pulse, about once each second. Settle into this as your basic awake state, a state of sensation without outside thoughts. Keep thoughts out. Sense only the pulse too slow for words. Let your eyes make small circles in time with your pulse, and with each pulse, drop into the sensation of your shoulders... of your upper arms... your lower arms... your hands. The sensation of your neck... your upper back... your lower back. The sensation of your chest... your stomach... your gut... your pelvis... your hips... your thighs... your knees... your calves... your ankles... and your feet. There is a lot to explore. Take it one step at a time.

Thoughtless sensations, awake and aware of your body's feelings. Not yet responsive to what's happening around you, not yet alert beyond listening and looking, looking out of a fog. Now we'll speed up, and as we speed up, watch how a curtain rises, and you find yourself on stage, in the act, in the round, all around you.

As the tempo rises, find yourself waking up more, engaging with a finer texture, more verbal, more inquisitive, attentive, furtive, and alert. There's a quarter note buried in the pulse, our first level of alertness. The quarter note of basic attention.

There is nothing special in the world about this frequency, but there is in us. It's the clock speed of broad thinking, the speed of basic talking, natural talking, and a common movement. Remember it in the rotation of your joints walking down a city sidewalk, sense it in the joints of other people walking down a city sidewalk. Some faster cities: New York or Tokyo. Some much slower: Venice, Italy or Kingston, Jamaica.

One, two, three, four... Automatic movement, robot attention, programmed limbs, our basic dance speed. You can drive or walk at this tempo, make breakfast, or sort the mail. Feel it in your eyes, a comfortable tension in your arms, an electric energy, a pressure bouncing like a wave between your wrists and your biceps. You're ready, engaged, focused on the ripples on the surface of wakefulness.

This is the rhythm of basic attention, but alertness wants more, a faster click, a smooth shifting of gears, but not just this. This is not enough. It gets old, boring, and dull in its incessant beat. It lacks novelty, both having surprise and reacting to it. A snap, a click, a spring, a trigger, a fuse, gunpowder kept dry and loaded. A laser awareness: discernment, armed to react.

Alertness combines three speeds that are happening at the same time. It's got polyrhythms, like music. There are always at least three. An awake speed gives you presence, a faster aware speed is engagement, and the fastest speed of being armed and ready, responding like a reflex. There are at least these three: present, engaged, and ready to react.

This faster speed is not persistent, not constant. If it were constant, we'd become deaf to it. It must be intermittent. You can feel it in the background, a back beat, a syncopation, like a fuse or trigger. It's not an action but a reaction, not a plateau but a jump. You have it reserved but only engage it on occasion. It keeps you armed and discerning. It keeps you mixed in motion. Otherwise you'll settle into a robot trance, and we often do settle into trance, but that's for sleep, not staying awake.

Now you're awake... One... Two... Three... Feel your pulse on each inhale, moving you forward like a stroke of the oars, your lungs creaking like the oar locks. Row! Beat... Beat... Beat... Beat. Row! Beat... Beat... Beat... Beat. There is no exertion.

Clear lungs of air wake you up, and your heart pumps awakeness through your torso, into your head, down your arms and legs, and into your hands and feet. You are awake, present, and listening. Lay it out like a base layer, like an undercoat, a foundation. You're in control.

Wake up… Get up… Hiccup… Imagine you're an eagle, and the air vibrates beneath your wings. Laid out flat, air pressing against your skin. Hear these beats in the land below you, in the cushion of air beneath you, in the heat rising, circling and soaring. Hear the rhythm in the land, alive.

Wake up… Get up… Rise up… Imagine you're a horse, and the solid earth vibrates below your pounding hooves. Muscles like spring boards, rebounding a polyrhythm on your spine, compression on a spring, waves. The drum head of the earth, played with your feet, echo and resonance. Resistance and resilience.

Swallow the rhythm into your being. You can feel the beats in the timing. Take the tempo into your tissues, a stretching in your sinuses, into the texture of your pulse, into the strike of your muscles, the tension of your tendons, the vibrations across and beneath your skin, across the fascia and the membranes.

Entrain these beats into your awareness, into your brain and its electricity; tempos buried under thoughts you ride, which carry you atop awareness: attentive, responsive. An eagle on the wing, a horse of the hoof, and the person of your mind.

Place these tempos in your hands and feet. Play them in your fine motor muscles. Store them in your muscle memory from where you can always retrieve them. Let them sink into your muscles like oil into thirsty wood, turning it golden and translucent. You are golden and translucent.

Whenever your alertness flags, feel the oil texture of your attentive rhythms. Lubricate your action and reaction to be audible again. It takes a few seconds, but you can do it. Whenever next you're tired, begin the unwrapping of these tempos and textures. Bring yourself back to tempo and rhythm without effort or strain.

Let the warm, liquid energy drain off you like warm water evaporating on a hot, dry day. Replace your awareness of the world around you, this day,

The Path to Sleep

this room, this time. Counting up, One... Two... Three... Back to now, feeling clear, able to recall and rebuild alertness with the simple, rhythmic tapping of your fingertips.

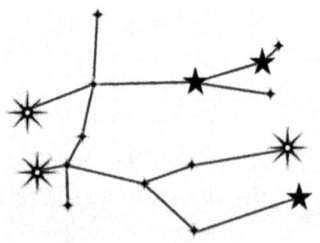

Hypnotic Session 24

Invitation

Audio file at: https://www.mindstrengthbalance.com/path-to-sleep-audio/

Take a deep breath, and sink into relaxation. Sink into that halfway state we've visited so much, halfway between presence and absence. Aware of your body, quiet in your mind, open in your feelings.

Take a stairway ten steps up to an elevated garden, a garden in the air. And as we take these steps to higher ground, feel the world fall away as the horizon sinks below us. The sky grows big as its color turns from cyan, to navy, to dark blue, and finally, when we reach the tenth step, to black.

One.

Two. Take a deep, easy breath.

Three.

Four. Let it out and relax like steam on a winter day.

Five.

Six. Open to those creatures that control the sky.

Seven.

Eight. To float up, into the air, where the plants reach.

Nine.

Ten. Into a thin black sky, under a blazing sun.

I'd like you to relax in a different way. I'd like you first to recognize who it is that relaxes, and have them sit within you separately, beside you. I'd like you to look at yourself as you have been all these years. Look at that constant part that has always been you, that has hardly changed since you were six. At least you know it's the same you now as then, even if others don't. That's who you are.

I'd like to ask you, who is it that wants to be more than you are now, or have been? I'd like to speak to that part of you that wishes you were

The Path to Sleep

something more, or something different, or would feel more comfortable if you lived in a different place or time.

If there is a part of you that knows what I mean, please ask that part of you to come forward comfortably, and give it space to do that, and accept it and its wishes, for now, and without judgment.

This part of you is natural, valuable, and wise. Ask this part of you to stay with us and stay beside us through this exercise. Let this part of you know that we will hear it without prejudice and honor its role and goals. Let this part please take my left hand so that I am beside you.

Now I'd like to ask you, who is it that wants things to be stable and supportive, to stay as they are, and to grow and mature?—and for that part of you to come forward, to make themselves present without hesitation and without any judgment on anyone's part. And this part of you is natural, too, and valuable, and wise.

Ask this part of you to stay with us through this exercise. Accept this voice that is yours, that is you, without criticism or hesitation. Let them have space, respect, and honor because that is their due. Let this part please take my right hand so that, again, I am beside you. I am beside both of you, between you, holding a hand of both.

These are two people of different inclination, two points of view, but they are more than that. They are two guides down two paths that would have led you differently had you listened to one and not the other. But you broker both, and take their direction to make them proud in alternation, but you also exasperate them as they sometimes are ignored. You think you can be judge and jury, balancing the happy middle road? You really can't expect to follow both, not as long as they're different people.

What do you have? What have you wrought for yourself?

I turn to my left hand, to that you who has dreamed so large and wanted so much more. Are they courageous or foolish, and how much have you followed them? And how do you feel about it? Never mind. I don't want your opinion. I want theirs.

I turn to them, and I ask them to tell you, in their own voice, of all that you could be and might yet become. What have you wrought for yourself?

Look to this person to discern the texture of risk and adventure. In whose company do they incline you? What are the tempos in those people who are packed to travel, who pull up their stakes like yesterday's vegetables? Do adventurers make you nervous? Do you feel comfortable around them?

When following your adventure, what is your mix of frequencies? How do you listen, act, and react? Where is your resistance? What is your vibe, your exuberance, your ponderance?

I turn to my right hand and that you that builds the stable, supportive, and sensible you. The you that plans for the future you think most likely. This is your practical side, but more than just a side, it is a person, with loves and lives, with private thoughts and secret feelings.

Pragmatic and practical, but frightened, too. Admit it. You give them more power than circumstances warrant. So few of our fears ever come to pass, navigating a river of phantoms most of whom we never meet because they never were.

When following your reasonable and practical self, what is your presentation? Who are you that feels comfortable among your peers of similarly reasonable and practical guides and guidesses? What are your vibrations? What places in your body encourage you to remain with the comfortable? What kind of people-energy makes you uncomfortable, or better said, who makes your practical self comfortable?

Now, I would like both of these people to let you go, and while I continue to hold their hands, I'd like you to drift out of their bodies into some other tones, some tones that are both higher and lower than the frequencies of either of your two guides.

And as I do, I'd like you to grow larger, break your earthen dam of friends and familiars, and let in the stranger, the traveler, the hermit, and grandmother.

The Path to Sleep

Let fall away your familiar frequencies of both of you, rhythms and tempos between which you've made most of your decisions, and take these two as a vibrating sound bath of greater visions and grander frequencies.

Drop your dichotomy of decisions, your duality of adventure or restraint, and replace their boundaries with something quite different.

Replace your familiar low frequency of extensions with this note that's even lower, and as it's lower, it's wider and longer. It takes in more and is more durable. A bigger space, a richer place, a vast space lit only by tea lights. An encounter of another kind, and let it resonate in you and make you grow bigger.

Replace your high frequencies, your discernments and reactions, your judgments and reflections, with these even higher frequencies, higher and ringing to the point of celestial. Perhaps too thin to breath, too ringing to remember, but let them resound nonetheless to entrain you.

Let it be clear in order to understand and accept the most distant and unlikely of events and possibilities, hopes, dreams, and the most enduring of rewards, the most meaningful and otherwise impossible, or maybe not impossible when tuned to a pitch this high. Open these vertical spaces, higher than the sky you thought was the limit.

Let these tones, the high and the low, break into your otherwise familiar frequencies of adventure and stability. Let these tones, the highs and the lows, be the apex of a triangle, whose two base angles are the two yous whose hands I hold: the evolver at my left and the preserver at my right.

With these higher high tones and lower low tones, call from within yourself another you, a greater visionary to see beyond the sky you've known and deeper in the firmament than you've thought possible. The frightening possibility that you might be more than you ever thought you could be and be secure and content with far less.

With their free hands, let the two yous whose hands I hold reach out to this transcendent vision, to clasp one of this visionary's hands in each of theirs, and so we form a circle, the three of you and me. Your two familiars

Wakefulness

both connected to the visionary, who is made of frequencies that were before outside your range.

Let them all come together now, all merge together. The adventurer, the protector, and the visionary who is resplendent. Molt the shells that limited your size before, and grow into these bigger spaces. Let all of them listen to each other with curious attention. Let each ask the other, more earnestly than before, what can each do for each other to make your goals realized for the continued betterment of you? You who are the democratically decided re-presentation of them.

You will work better with the poles of your own dichotomy, but much more than that. You will work beyond the poles of your dichotomy, going further and perpendicular to hear the music of higher spheres and become yourself a transmitter of insight, transformation, and potential to those around you, who came before you, and who come after.

With this, let our small group of four merge into two: you and I. And return to now and here. Back from the black sky garden, to the steps down to the firmament of blues and greens and yellows.

The world we take for granted is not the limit of your potential any more than you are limited to mold upon its surface. You have elevation, and you have feet. Let the ringing in our ears remind us of how much more we can always be.

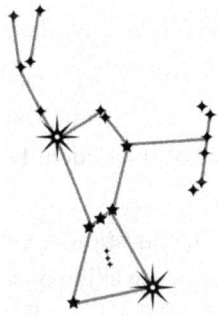

13 Epilogue

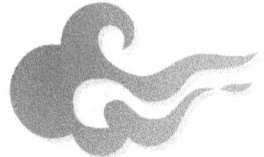

EXPANDING OUR LIMITS.

Are we limited in our understanding to only those things that we can turn into a story or put into words? Can we have a bigger understanding of who we are and what issues define us than the stories we tell?

Our understanding is limited by our language if we limit our thinking to it. But there are things that are like language, that have a greater scope than any language we speak, and those "things" are our bodies and imaginations.

If we break out of the structure of stories, with their focus on sequence, character, and will, and embrace our unbounded imaginations, then we find ourselves free of time, identity, and goal.

If we break out of the structure of our egos, which focus on constructions, presentations, reactions, and expectations, and immerse ourselves in the cacophony of sensation, then we find ourselves directly connected to a dynamic web of actions bigger, smaller, more, and less complex than ourselves.

The realm of the body and the realm of dreams offer an infinitely larger palette with which to paint an understanding of the world. You might say that these palettes are the world and that you are the brush that paints what you see.

Why be limited? There are a million reasons and arguments for each of them, and it's a swamp, and you're lost in it. You're always lost in it because, in fact, the world does operate free of time, identity, and goals, and we can't, at least not always.

There is some symmetry in the questions we can ask of all our worlds. Ask these questions of your sleeping and waking consciousnesses:

- How do you know when you're dreaming? How do you know if you're awake?
- Is your lack of control in your dreams all that different from your lack of control in your waking life?

Ask these questions of your body. Your body speaks slowly and not necessarily when you're listening, so listen over time.

- Who is setting the limits of your capability, and can you change these?
- Is your lack of control over your body all that different from your lack of control of your world?
- If you changed your perception of rates of time and space, would your body also change?

Just as we need a chemical atmosphere to breathe, we need a conceptual atmosphere to think. Your ego is your spaceship. It is part of your vehicle. It is your perception of mind and body, and it guides you places, but it's not all you are.

You have problems sleeping, so you say. Your vehicle isn't working, and you don't know what to do. Your spaceship is smart—smarter than you are, I hope—and it knows how to fix itself, but it needs a reason. Stop kicking, shouting, and grinding the ignition. Maybe it's not broken. Maybe you are.

Your vehicle will fix itself once it knows it can trust you. Be a responsible driver. Find your purpose. Find the parking lot, the overlook, the beach, the trail head. Park your ego. Get out. Gather your essentials, and head off into the desert, the woods, the mountains, the lakes, or the wilderness. Sail off across the sea. You'll sleep better for it.

"You have to go on and be crazy. Craziness is like heaven."
— Jimi Hendrix (1942—1970)

THE END

Appendix: Alphabetical List of Air Filtering House Plants

Aloe vera, leaves are a skin salve, filters formaldehyde, tolerant.

Bamboo palm (Chamaedorea seifritzii), filters formaldehyde.

Boston fern (Nephrolepis exaltata), effective oxygenator and humidifier.

Chinese evergreen (Aglaonema modestum), oxygenator/purifier.

Dracaena, filters xylene, formaldehyde, benzene, and trichloroethylene, but toxic if eaten by pets.

Garden mum (Chrysanthemum morifolium), removes building material toxins formaldehyde, ammonia, benzene, and xylene.

Gerbera daisy (Gerbera jamesonii), purifies and boosts oxygen at night.

Golden pothos (Epipiremnum aureum), oxygenator/purifier.

Heartleaf philodendron (Philodendron scandens), oxygenator/purifier.

Japanese royal fern (Osmunda japonica), filters formaldehyde.

Peace lily (Spathiphyllum), fragrant, filters trichloroethylene, benzene, ammonia, and formaldehyde, hearty and shade tolerant.

Snake plant (Sansevieria trifasciata) very drought and low-light tolerant, filters trichloroethylene, benzene, xylene, and formaldehyde.

Spider plant (Chlorophytum comosum) very drought but needs bright, indirect sunlight. Filters xylene and formaldehyde.

Weeping fig (Fiscus benjamina) drought and low-light tolerant, filters benzene and formaldehyde, produces fruits and grows up to ten feet.

References

Lewis, Marc D. (2005). "Bridging Emotion Theory and Neurobiology Through Dynamic Systems Modeling." In *Behavioral and Brain Sciences*, 28(2), pp. 169–245.

McGuire, William and Hull, R.F.C. (Eds.) (1977). *C.G. Jung Speaking: Interviews and Encounters*. Princeton University Press, Princeton, NJ, p. 419.

Pinker, Steven (2003). "Language as an Adaptation to the Cognitive Niche," in M. Christiansen and S. Kirby (Eds.) *Language Evolution: States of the Art*. Oxford University Press, New York, NY, pp. 16-37.

Suddendorf, T., Addis, D. R., and Corballis, M. C. (2009). "Mental Time Travel and The Shaping of the Human Mind," in *Philosophical Transactions of the Royal Society*, B, 364(1521), pp. 1317-1324.

Taylor, Shelley E. (2011). "Envisioning the Future and Self-Regulation," in M. Bar (Ed.) *Predictions in the Brain: Using Our Past to Prepare for the Future*, Oxford University Press, New York, NY, pp. 134-143.

Tedlock, Barbara (1991). "The New Anthropology of Dreaming," in *Dreaming*, 1(2), pp. 161-178.

Tholey, Paul (1983). "Techniques for Inducing and Manipulating Lucid Dreams," in *Perceptual and Motor Skills*, 57(1), pp.79-90.

Tholey, Paul (1988). "A Model for Lucidity Training, as a Means of Self-healing and Psychological Growth," in J. Gackenbail, and S. LaBerge (Eds.), *Conscious Mind, Sleeping Brain*. Plenum Press, New York, NY, pp. 263-290.

Thorne, Kip S. (1994). *Black Holes and Time Warps, Einstein's Outrageous Legacy*. W.W. Norton & Co. New York, NY, p. 462.

Bibliography

Barrett, Deirdre (2001). *The Committee of Sleep: How Artists, Scientists, and Athletes Use Their Dreams for Creative Problem Solving—and How You Can Too.* Crown Publishers, New York, NY.

Blum, Ralph H. (1993). *The Book of Runes.* St. Martin's Press, New York, NY.

Davidow, Jenny (2012). *Embracing Your Subconscious: Bringing All Parts of You Into Creative Partnership.* Tidal Wave Press.

Feldenkrais, Moshe (2011). *Embodied Wisdom: The Collected Papers of Moshe Feldenkrais.* North Atlantic Books, Berkeley, CA.

LaBerge, Stephen (2009). *Lucid Dreaming: A Concise Guide to Awakening in Your Dreams and in Your Life.* Sounds True, Boulder, CO.

Rosenberg, Robert S. (2014). *Sleep Soundly Every Night, Feel Fantastic Every Day: A Doctor's Guide to Solving Your Sleep Problems.* Demos Health Publishing, New York, NY.

Walker, Matthew (2017). *Why We Sleep, Unlocking the Power of Sleep and Dreams.* Simon and Schuster, New York, NY.

Wangyal, Tenzin (1998). *The Tibetan Yogas Of Dream And Sleep.* Snow Lion, Ithaca, NY.

About the Author

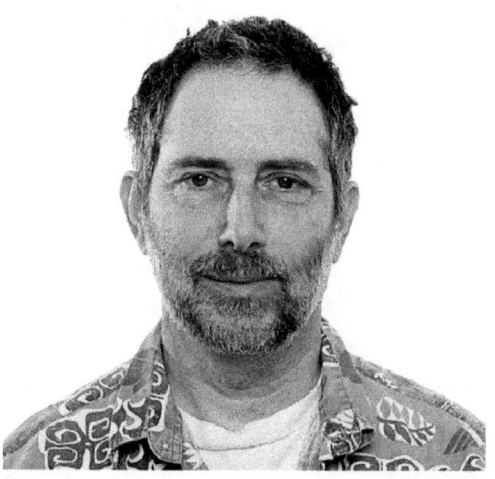

As a child, Lincoln Stoller joined his family on extended foreign vacations, traveled across the USA as his father's photo assistant, and left his suburban New York neighborhood as soon as he could stick out his thumb. Drawn to the mountains of Europe and North American, his travels opened him to alternative states of mind as well as European, Hispanic, African, and indigenous cultures.

After studying physics at a half dozen colleges, working as an astronomer at the University of California at Berkeley, and getting a PhD in quantum physics at the University of Texas at Austin, he spent two decades creating business software. Then, following his interest in music, a series of unlikely events led to mentorships in brainwave biofeedback, his certification as a hypnotherapist, and publications in the fields of neurofeedback, hypnotherapy, psychology, and neuroscience.

His first book, *The Learning Project, Rites of Passage*, explores the role of learning in how people create a meaningful life. His second book, *Becoming Lucid, Self-Awareness in Sleeping & Waking Life*, is both an exploration of and a tutorial on how to achieve lucidity. *The Path to Sleep* is his third book.

Lincoln works as a therapist and consultant to individuals and businesses and publishes in a diversity of fields. His two exceptional sons are close in heart, but separated by age and distance on opposite sides of the continent. Lincoln currently resides in the city of Victoria, British Columbia, Canada.

www.ingramcontent.com/pod-product-compliance
Lightning Source LLC
Chambersburg PA
CBHW051540020426
42333CB00016B/2022